# ONCOLOGY NURSE NAVIGATION
# CASE STUDIES

**Edited by**
Penny Daugherty, RN, MS, OCN®
Kathleen A. Gamblin, RN, BSN, OCN®
Margaret Rummel, RN, MHA, OCN®, NE-BC

Oncology Nursing Society
Pittsburgh, Pennsylvania

**ONS Publications Department**
Publisher and Director of Publications: William A. Tony, BA, CQIA
Managing Editor: Lisa M. George, BA
Assistant Managing Editor: Amy Nicoletti, BA, JD
Acquisitions Editor: John Zaphyr, BA, MEd
Copy Editors: Vanessa Kattouf, BA, Andrew Petyak, BA
Graphic Designer: Dany Sjoen
Editorial Assistant: Judy Holmes

### Library of Congress Cataloging-in-Publication Data

Names: Daugherty, Penny, editor. | Gamblin, Kathleen A., editor. | Rummel, Margaret A., editor. | Oncology Nursing Society, issuing body.
Title: Oncology nurse navigation case studies / edited by Penny Daugherty, Kathleen A. Gamblin, Margaret Rummel.
Other titles: Complemented by (work): Oncology nurse navigation.
Description: Pittsburgh, Pennsylvania : Oncology Nursing Society, [2016] | Complemented by: Oncology nurse navigation / edited by Karyl D. Blaseg, Penny Daugherty, and Kathleen A. Gamblin. 2014. | Includes bibliographical references.
Identifiers: LCCN 2016042539 | ISBN 9781935864936
Subjects: | MESH: Oncology Nursing–methods | Patient Navigation–methods | Nurse's Role | Case Reports
Classification: LCC RC266 | NLM WY 156 | DDC 616.99/40231–dc23 LC record available at https://lccn.loc.gov/2016042539

### Publisher's Note

This book is published by the Oncology Nursing Society (ONS). ONS neither represents nor guarantees that the practices described herein will, if followed, ensure safe and effective patient care. The recommendations contained in this book reflect ONS's judgment regarding the state of general knowledge and practice in the field as of the date of publication. The recommendations may not be appropriate for use in all circumstances. Those who use this book should make their own determinations regarding specific safe and appropriate patient care practices, taking into account the personnel, equipment, and practices available at the hospital or other facility at which they are located. The editors and publisher cannot be held responsible for any liability incurred as a consequence from the use or application of any of the contents of this book. Figures and tables are used as examples only. They are not meant to be all-inclusive, nor do they represent endorsement of any particular institution by ONS. Mention of specific products and opinions related to those products do not indicate or imply endorsement by ONS. Websites mentioned are provided for information only; the hosts are responsible for their own content and availability. Unless otherwise indicated, dollar amounts reflect U.S. dollars.

ONS publications are originally published in English. Publishers wishing to translate ONS publications must contact ONS about licensing arrangements. ONS publications cannot be translated without obtaining written permission from ONS. (Individual tables and figures that are reprinted or adapted require additional permission from the original source.) Because translations from English may not always be accurate or precise, ONS disclaims any responsibility for inaccuracies in words or meaning that may occur as a result of the translation. Readers relying on precise information should check the original English version.

Printed in the United States of America

Innovation • Excellence • Advocacy

# Contributors

## Editors

**Penny Daugherty, RN, MS, OCN®**
Gynecologic Oncology Nurse Navigator
Northside Hospital Cancer Institute
Atlanta, Georgia
*Case 8. Developing a Relationship With a*
*Newly Diagnosed Patient*

**Kathleen A. Gamblin, RN, BSN, OCN®**
Oncology Patient Navigation Coordinator
Northside Hospital Cancer Institute
Atlanta, Georgia
*Case 1. Establishing a Navigation Program*
*in a Statewide Multifacility System;*
*Case 11. Lung Cancer*

**Margaret Rummel, RN, MHA, OCN®,**
**NE-BC**
Oncology Nurse Navigator
Abramson Cancer Center
Penn Medicine
Philadelphia, Pennsylvania
*Case 16. Navigating a Patient With*
*Multiple Disparities*

## Authors

**Robin Atkinson, RN, BSN, OCN®**
Gynecology Oncology Nurse Navigator
Novant Health Derrick L. Davis Cancer
Center
Winston-Salem, North Carolina
*Case 9. Cancer at a Young Age*

**Emily Mason Beard, RN, BSN, OCN®,**
**CBCN®**
Women's Oncology Program Coordinator
Northside Hospital Cancer Institute
Atlanta, Georgia
*Case 22. Oncology Nurse Navigator Inte-*
*gration Into the Multidisciplinary Care*
*Continuum*

**Debbie Bickes, RN, MN, OCN®**
Program Coordinator
Northside Hospital Cancer Institute
Atlanta, Georgia
*Case 2. Integrating Lay Navigators Within*
*an Existing Nurse Navigator Program*

**Tami Borneman, MSN, CNS, FPCN**
Senior Research Specialist
City of Hope
Duarte, California
*Case 18. Transitioning to Palliative Care*

**Frank dela Rama, RN, MS, AOCNS®, AGN-BC**
Clinical Nurse Specialist, Oncology/Genomics and Prostate Cancer Nurse Navigator
Palo Alto Medical Foundation
Palo Alto, California
*Case 13. Advanced Prostate Cancer*

**Betty Ferrell, PhD, RN, FAAN, FPCN**
Director of Nursing Research and Education
City of Hope
Duarte, California
*Case 18. Transitioning to Palliative Care*

**Barbara Francks, RN, BSN, OCN®, CBCN®**
Clinical Nurse Navigator
Sentara Williamsburg Regional Medical Center
Williamsburg, Virginia
*Case 7. Navigating a Young Patient*

**Sharon Gentry, RN, MSN, AOCN®, CBCN®**
Breast Nurse Navigator
Novant Health Derrick L. Davis Cancer Center
Winston-Salem, North Carolina
*Case 5. Breast Cancer in an Older Adult Patient*

**Alice S. Kerber, MN, APRN, ACNS-BC, AOCN®, AGN-BC**
Oncology and Genetics Nurse Specialist
Georgia Center for Oncology Research and Education (CORE)
Atlanta, Georgia
*Case 4. Ethics: Supporting the Family Journey*

**Venteria L. Knight, RN, MPH**
Patient Navigator, Oncology
Piedmont Healthcare
Stockbridge, Georgia
*Case 17. Overcoming the Financial and Emotional Barriers of Patients*

**Lori McMullen, RN, MSN, OCN®**
Clinical and Program Manager—Cancer Services
Matthews Center for Cancer Care, University Medical Center of Princeton at Plainsboro
Plainsboro, New Jersey
*Case 12. Genitourinary Cancer*

**Nicole Messier, RN, BSN, OCN®**
GI/GU Nurse Navigator and Clinical Program Coordinator
University of Vermont Medical Center
Burlington, Vermont
*Case 10. Rectal Cancer*

**Eleanor Miller, MSN, RN, OCN®, CBCN®**
Manager—Oncology Nurse Navigation
Abramson Cancer Center
Penn Medicine
Philadelphia, Pennsylvania
*Case 20. The Unexpected Caregiver*

**Elissa A. Peters, RN, MS, OCN®, CBCN®**
Breast Cancer Nurse Navigator
Penrose Cancer Center
Colorado Springs, Colorado
*Case 19. The Post-Treatment Phase*

**Paula Sanborn, RN, BSN, CPHON®**
Sarcoma Nurse Navigator
Nationwide Children's Hospital
Columbus, Ohio
*Case 14. Osteosarcoma and Mucositis in an Adolescent Patient; Case 15. Rhabdomyosarcoma in a Pediatric Patient*

**Amy Sebastian-Deutsch, DNP, APRN, CNS, AOCNS®**
Director of Oncology Services
Houston Methodist Sugar Land Hospital
Sugar Land, Texas
*Case 21. Navigator Collaboration*

**Jean B. Sellers, RN, MSN**
Administrative Clinical Director—University of North Carolina Cancer Network
University of North Carolina Lineberger Comprehensive Cancer Center
Chapel Hill, North Carolina
*Case 3. Increasing the Cancer Workforce With Lay Patient Navigation*

**Lillie D. Shockney, RN, BS, MAS**
University Distinguished Service Professor
  of Breast Cancer, Johns Hopkins Univer-
  sity School of Medicine, Departments of
  Surgery and Oncology
Administrative Director, Johns Hopkins
  University Breast Center
Director, Cancer Survivorship Programs
  at the Sidney Kimmel Comprehensive
  Cancer Center at Johns Hopkins
Professor, Johns Hopkins University
  School of Medicine, Departments of
  Surgery, Oncology, and Gynecology and
  Obstetrics
Adjunct Professor, Johns Hopkins Univer-
  sity School of Nursing
Baltimore, Maryland
*Case 6. Metastatic Breast Cancer*

**Anne Zobec, MS, AOCNP®, BC**
Oncology Nurse Practitioner
Rocky Mountain Cancer Centers
Colorado Springs, Colorado
*Case 19. The Post-Treatment Phase*

## Disclosure

Editors and authors of books and guidelines provided by the Oncology Nursing Society are expected to disclose to the readers any significant financial interest or other relationships with the manufacturer(s) of any commercial products.

A vested interest may be considered to exist if a contributor is affiliated with or has a financial interest in commercial organizations that may have a direct or indirect interest in the subject matter. A "financial interest" may include, but is not limited to, being a shareholder in the organization; being an employee of the commercial organization; serving on an organization's speakers bureau; or receiving research funding from the organization. An "affiliation" may be holding a position on an advisory board or some other role of benefit to the commercial organization. Vested interest statements appear in the front matter for each publication.

Contributors are expected to disclose any unlabeled or investigational use of products discussed in their content. This information is acknowledged solely for the information of the readers.

The contributors provided the following disclosure and vested interest information:

Margaret Rummel, RN, MHA, OCN®, NE-BC: Academy of Oncology Nurse Navigators, Millennium Pharmaceuticals, consultant or advisory role

Sharon Gentry, RN, MSN, AOCN®, CBCN®: Academy of Oncology Nurse Navigators, leadership position and honoraria; Genentech, consultant or advisory role; Pfizer, honoraria

Alice S. Kerber, MN, APRN, ACNS-BC, AOCN®, AGN-BC: Pfizer, honoraria

Lori McMullen, RN, MSN, OCN®: Haymarket Publishing, honoraria and other remuneration

Nicole Messier, RN, BSN, OCN®: Academy of Oncology Nurse Navigators, Teva Pharmaceuticals, honoraria

Jean B. Sellers, RN, MSN: North Carolina Oncology Navigator Association, leadership position; Haymarket Media, Lilly Oncology, consultant or advisory role; Pfizer, honoraria

Lillie D. Shockney, RN, BS, MAS: Pfizer Oncology, consultant or advisory role

Anne Zobec, MS, AOCNP®, BC: Amgen, Boehringer Ingelheim, Exelixis, Genentech, honoraria

# Contents

# Preface

This book is meant to serve as a companion to the Oncology Nursing Society (ONS) publication *Oncology Nurse Navigation: Delivering Patient-Centered Care Across the Continuum* (2014), which explored the building of programs and individual disease-specific sites. We have refined this approach in the pages that follow, focusing on individual navigators using skilled guidance in patient-centric scenarios.

All books tell a story. This one has many to share. Through varying case studies, navigators from across the country have generously contributed their individual experiences with patients (and caregivers) in guiding them through their cancer diagnoses and treatments.

It is our hope that these studies will not only provide education and resources for our readers, but also showcase the diverse roles and challenges navigators face in facilitating access to treatment, alleviating numerous care barriers, and providing support, resources, and education throughout the disease trajectory.

This is a "snippet" of what navigators do, and we are well aware that significant advances are being made in our field. Navigators must be at the top of their game and able to think "outside the box" as we traverse the cancer experience with our patients and their loved ones sharing the journey.

This book chronicles the development of several successful navigation programs, including the following:

- One large urban hospital system, which burgeoned from an oncology nurse navigator model on the main campus into a multisite enduring initiative, incorporating lay navigators and nurse navigators providing multifaceted care for patients in 12 statewide locations
- A metropolitan lay navigation program, which enhanced care immeasurably to its residents
- An amazing statewide program, spearheaded by one nurse navigator, which provided outreach to its barrier islands

We hope that the stories of these individual programs will provide inspiration to those wanting to initiate their own navigation programs.

Our overarching goal is to provide a comprehensive anthology from all around the United States, touching on as many disease sites as possible. As we brainstormed about the case studies to be featured, we were fortunate to include the perspective of a pediatric nurse navigator—a unique role that many of us will never experience. Alas, as one of our field reviewers pointed out, we missed a case study specifically touching on the special needs of the older adult population. As with all education, opportunity for growth always exists.

In designing this book, we were ever mindful that ONS is evaluating "role delineation and standards of practice." Our hope is that certification within the field of oncology nurse navigation will be developed. To this end, each author has included evidence-based questions at the conclusion of each case study.

Navigation plays a crucial role in patient care. It is recognized as a basic component of oncology care and is mandated by the American College of Surgeons Commission on Cancer (CoC). All CoC organizations are expected to be able to speak to the art and science of navigation. We are in an exponentially evolving field, and our hope is that this book will help fill some of the existing knowledge gaps.

The editors would like to recognize the many authors who worked long and hard in writing these case studies, which will benefit a wide range of readers.

We thank our families, friends, and colleagues. Without your support and guidance, this book would not have come to fruition.

We thank ONS for believing in us and the ONS Publications Department for guiding us on this adventure.

We also thank our patients for allowing us to be a part of their journeys. It has been our privilege to be a part of this with them. We have learned so much from every patient!

It is our hope that you, the reader, will benefit from the many years of navigation experience that the authors have shared and apply the information learned from their navigation roles.

Penny Daugherty, RN, MS, OCN®
Kathleen A. Gamblin, RN, BSN, OCN®
Margaret Rummel, RN, MHA, OCN®, NE-BC

# Foreword

*Oncology Nurse Navigation Case Studies* describes the special contributions to patient care made by oncology nurse navigators who manage patients with site-specific cancers and work with lay navigation programs. This book builds on a previous Oncology Nursing Society publication, *Oncology Nurse Navigation: Delivering Patient-Centered Care Across the Continuum* (2014).

In 1990, I introduced the patient navigation concept and model at Harlem Hospital Center in New York, New York, as an attempt in diminishing the extremely high breast cancer death rate in a population of poor black women. Studies over two time periods showed that the combined interventions of breast cancer screening and patient navigation dramatically improved the five-year breast cancer survival rate of this population (from 39% to 70%). From this origin, patient navigation has become widely adopted in the nation as a strategy to improve cancer outcomes, particularly among the medically underserved.

Significant markers of this national progress include the signing of the Patient Navigator Outreach and Chronic Disease Prevention Act by President George W. Bush in 2005 and the American College of Surgeons Commission on Cancer (CoC) mandate in 2015, which stated that patient navigation is a standard of care required for cancer center approval. Currently, more than 1,500 cancer centers in the United States are approved by CoC. Yet, to gain an understanding of the progress we have made in patient navigation, it may be helpful to reflect on what conditions led to the patient navigation concept and model.

In my early experiences as a cancer surgeon at Harlem Hospital Center in the 1970s, more than half of my patients had advanced breast cancer at the time of initial treatment. Some women presented with ulcerated masses. I found ways to provide free breast cancer screenings. These screenings helped, but many women with abnormal findings had very long delays before treatment. So I focused on navigating patients (eliminating barriers to timely diagnosis) from the point of abnormal finding to diagnostic resolution. Later, these services were expanded to patient navigation across the healthcare continuum, which encompasses outreach, screening, detection, diagnosis, treatment, and post-treatment quality-of-life support.

I wish to underscore the following conclusions:

- We must seek to provide high-quality treatment (and navigation, as needed) to all patients with a cancer diagnosis. Particularly in poor and underserved communities, it is important to begin patient navigation before a cancer diagnosis—for example, at the point of abnormal finding. This is because the dominant cause of higher cancer mortality is late-stage disease at the time of initial treatment.

- Accomplishing this requires a team approach, which includes both professional and lay navigators. The type of navigator depends on the navigation phase. Oncology nurse navigators are best prepared to navigate patients with a cancer diagnosis.

- Lay navigators can best assist by eliminating financial, communication, and medical system barriers faced by patients both in the community and in the course of diagnosis and treatment.

*Oncology Nurse Navigation Case Studies* illustrates how oncology nurse navigators are expanding the scope of oncology nursing within and across cancer specialties. This publication also presents case studies showing effective collaboration between oncology nurse navigators and lay navigation programs, illustrating how oncology nurse navigators have become leaders in the evolving field of patient navigation.

Harold P. Freeman, MD
Founder and President
Harold P. Freeman Patient Navigation Institute

# Establishing a Navigation Program in a Statewide Multifacility System

Kathleen A. Gamblin, RN, BSN, OCN®

The following two case studies reflect the development of oncology nurse navigation and lay navigation, both of which were successfully integrated in a program at the Northside Hospital Cancer Institute (NHCI). NHCI is a community cancer program serving the Atlanta metropolitan area. This program includes three acute care hospitals and two affiliated medical oncology practices spanning 32 offices across 29 counties in northern and central Georgia.

The Oncology Patient Navigation Program was initiated in 2010 with NHCI's participation in the National Cancer Institute Community Cancer Centers Program (NCCCP). This navigation program began with four hospital-based oncology nurse navigators (ONNs). After six years, that number grew to 25, including 15 ONNs and 10 lay navigators. These navigators cover not only the three hospitals within the system, but also 13 offices of the affiliated medical oncology practices. Program management and strategic planning are centralized under the oversight of an oncology patient navigation program coordinator, who ensures consistency and uniformity across the system, allowing for coordinated, systematic growth of the program.

## What methods were used to assess the need for and structure of the navigation program?

From the inception of navigation at NHCI, the intent was to build a formalized navigation program with a leadership and supervisory structure, rather than simply adding navigators and having no dedicated leadership. To ensure the program's success, it was important to understand the navigation processes already present in the organization and evaluate all areas of the oncology continuum.

A gap analysis is the first step in designing and building any navigation program (Mack & Shalkowski, 2014). At NHCI, this assessment was conducted by key personnel and physicians in the oncology continuum to identify areas where navigation potentially could be valuable. Information was thoroughly evaluated in a community needs assessment, which included identified areas of focus by the hospital system as well as data from the cancer registry regarding volumes in specific tumor types.

Mack and Shalkowski (2014) emphasized the importance of a "systematic design, using qualitative and quantitative information to gain insight for program development" (p. 50). To this end, a literature search on navigation was completed, and information was gathered on other navigation programs throughout the country via site visits, phone calls, and emails to key personnel. The information obtained from these steps was used in building the program.

As with any new role in health care, the ONN role at NHCI was surrounded by questions. For example, how was the ONN role different than that of the oncology social worker, the case management staff, or even other oncology nurses in the system?

Although a preliminary job description was written at the onset of the program, it became apparent that additional work was necessary to redraft this description to further characterize this distinctive role.

## How was the role of the ONN differentiated from other roles within the NHCI program?

Early in NHCI's literature search on navigation, information was obtained on the implementation of the navigation role in Canada. The country's publicly funded system enabled oncology navigation to become implemented and studied, leading to the development of literature about its programs. Of particular interest to NHCI was a professional navigation framework validated in a Canadian context. Fillion et al. (2012) felt that the literature failed to describe cancer navigation consistently and that confusion over the role was related to the "lack of acknowledgment of the bidimensional nature of the role" (p. E58). This bidimensional role consisted of a health system–oriented first dimension focusing on the continuity of care of the patient and a patient-centered second dimension focusing on patient empowerment. This framework most closely matched NHCI's goals of moving the patient through the system efficiently and meeting the patient's psychosocial needs.

The Supportive Care Framework for Cancer Care also was used as a foundation in the implementation and delivery of navigation services. Formulated by Fitch in 1994, this framework was "designed as a tool for cancer care professionals and program managers to conceptualize what type of help cancer patients might require and how planning for service delivery might be approached" (Fitch, 2008, p. 6).

When evolved into practice, these frameworks helped to differentiate the ONN role and build the theoretical foundation for the NHCI program.

Finally, core competencies developed by the National Coalition of Oncology Nurse Navigators and the Oncology Nursing Society (ONS) were used to fill specific functions and outline the job description of the ONN role.

These competencies and their development were critical for two reasons. First, they prevented the ONN role from becoming defined by assigned "tasks." Many times, the tasks of the navigator became so numerous and unrelated to the role that the potential positive influence on the patient was lessened (Advisory Board Company, 2011). Second, they ensured that the ONN role had a specific scope of practice moving forward, as the lay navigation component was added.

NHCI wanted to avoid a duplication of services among the navigation team (nurse and lay) and confusion among the healthcare system staff and patients. Although some overlap inevitably would occur, enough delineation was present to ensure that all navigators understood their role.

To further differentiate the two, lay navigation team members were called *cancer care liaisons* (CCLs). In the Oncology Patient Navigation Program, the role of the disease site navigator is reserved for ONNs who have clinical expertise, while the CCLs function as support and provide both system and community resources for patients.

The program's initial launch began with a program coordinator and four ONNs in the sites of breast, lung, gynecology, and gastrointestinal tumors. These sites were decided based on information obtained from the cancer registry related to total patient volume at NHCI.

## How were the actual processes of navigation developed for the tumor-specific sites?

Prior to the initiation of the navigation program, a national consulting firm advised in its early development and outlined a process for ONNs to receive referrals for patients from NHCI's oncology registry pathology reporting system; however, during the gap analysis, it was determined that working through this system might actually lead to delays in identifying oncology patients needing navigation. Further surveys were conducted in each of the sites to determine how patients moved through the disease continuum and what providers, clinicians, and others involved in patient care viewed as the best initial entry point of navigation as well as potential points of navigator intervention. From this, processes and written algorithms were developed.

With this framework in place, so began the process of continual evaluation and change based on the needs of patients, caregivers, and the system. The NCCCP Navigation Assessment Tool was used not only to provide a baseline assessment of the navigation program as a whole, but also to establish algorithms within the individual disease site programs. The tool also was used in the development of future goals in each of the disease sites (Swanson, Strusowski, Mack, & Degroot, 2012).

Each program functioned in slightly different ways. The breast ONNs received their referrals from the positive pathology reports of patients who were biopsied at Northside Hospital. The gynecologic ONNs received referrals from mid-level providers assigned to the inpatient unit where patients were sent after surgery (as gynecology patients frequently are not positively diagnosed until the time of surgery). The thoracic ONNs most often received referrals for patients with a strong suspicion of lung cancer who also were undergoing diagnostic procedures. Although ONN functions were slightly different in each disease site, every patient encounter began with a standardized assessment developed for NHCI patients.

## Why is navigation assessment important?

ONNs are able to use their knowledge and skill to assess patients and identify potential barriers to care (Gentry & Sellers, 2014).

Assessment is important, as it provides a baseline for the ONN to formulate a plan to support and care for both patients and caregivers. Although no standardized navigation assessment exists, each program develops its own, adapts a model from another program, or uses other types of psychosocial screening.

The NHCI navigation program started with the development of a basic assessment tool based on adaptions from several other programs. After a period of initial use, it became apparent that further revision or the adaption of another assessment tool was needed. With further research, a navigation assessment was developed based on seven categories found in Fitch's (2008) framework: physical, informational, emotional, psychological, social, spiritual, and practical. These categories have allowed for more in-depth assessment and determination of patient and caregiver needs. Not only is information from this assessment used by the ONN, but it also is conveyed to a multidisciplinary conference coordinator to alert the multidisciplinary care team of any potential issues that may influence patient care and additional needs.

The initial expectation of the NHCI navigation program was that all patients would be navigated. It became increasingly apparent that this probably would not be possible based on a multitude of factors, including patient refusal of navigation, increasing analytic case volumes, patients diagnosed at NHCI but treated elsewhere, and patients who were not identified because of the many points of entry along the cancer continuum. The next section will address how to target patients most in need of navigation services.

## How are NHCI patients identified for navigation, and which patients most likely need navigation?

Patients in need of nurse navigation are identified by direct referral from physicians and staff; through multidisciplinary conferences, hospital census reports, surgery schedules, and screening programs; or from self-referral inside or outside the system. Regardless of how patients are identified, the concept of *patient-centered care*, where patients are "listened to, informed, respected, and involved in their care—and their wishes are honored," is applied first and foremost as an indispensable principle in the navigator program (Epstein & Street, 2011, p. 100).

Although the ONN, physician, or staff may think a patient requires navigation assistance, the patient may not feel that way. Navigation is offered as a service to patients, and patients always retain the right to refuse this service.

Fitch's (2008) framework, used in the development of the navigation program at NHCI, has basic clinical standards for the supportive care of patients with cancer. Two of these standards are significant in determining the process of referring patients to navigation.

The first standard states, "All individuals have the opportunity to be referred to an appropriate supportive care resource" (Fitch, 2008, p. 12). All NHCI patients should be given the opportunity to be referred to navigation. To this end, physicians and staff are educated about the services offered by navigation. A brochure and letter detailing the services of the navigation program are provided to the patients, along with a navigation-specific phone number and email address. In addition, navigation is highlighted on the NHCI website (www.northside .com/Oncology-Patient-Navigation) and through multiple print publications available to the community.

The second standard states, "All individuals have the opportunity for self-referral to supportive care resources" (Fitch, 2008, p. 12). ONNs proactively contact patients identified as needing navigation services. From that initial contact it is left to the patient to continue proactive contact or initiate contact at a later date. Patients who prefer to initiate contact need to be educated on available navigation services at any point along the cancer continuum. Determining the patients most likely to need navigation remains an ongoing discussion; patients who would seem to have the greatest need often do not use the navigation services, and patients with a seemingly low need may contact the navigator on a regular basis.

Currently, no validated acuity systems exist in navigation; however, the Billings Clinic in Montana developed an acuity system to help ensure a more standardized workload for each navigator (Blaseg, 2009). NHCI currently is working on an acuity scale that combines elements of the Billings system with characteristics of patients of higher need at NHCI. The hope is that this scale will allow for a more even distribution level of care and act as a guide to determine which patients require a more proactive, hands-on approach from navigation.

Since November 2010, NHCI has added ONNs in the new tumor type sites of melanoma/sarcoma, neurologic, general, and screening. It also has added additional ONNs in lung and breast.

NHCI also has participated in the Centers for Medicare and Medicaid's Health Care Innovation Challenge Awards grant as a Cancer Care Network affiliate of the University of Alabama at Birmingham, adding lay navigation to the system. This program has added six staff to NHCI's navigation program. After the initial year of the grant, it was recognized that lay navigators (or CCLs) could further delineate their role on the NHCI navigation program team. The greatest need was found to be in the affiliated medical oncology offices. A pilot project was initiated with one CCL in one medical oncology practice. This project has since expanded to an additional five CCLs serving eight affiliated medical oncology practices.

## How does the CCL function in medical oncology practices?

Although many functions exist in navigation, not every function requires a trained oncology nurse; thus, the lay navigator role was created. Common questions asked within NHCI include the following:
- What is the current need?
- Who is the best person to meet that need?

For example, a nurse does not necessarily need to be making appointments or coordinating transportation. A CCL with these areas of expertise might enhance the experience between the patient and caregiver.

Medical oncology practices most often are staffed with RNs with expertise in oncology who already provide the clinical teaching, symptom management, and care coordination roles. The CCL job function and description was developed with input from physicians, nurses, and clinic managers, along with the core competencies for non–clinically licensed patient navigators created by the George Washington University Cancer Institute (Pratt-Chapman, Willis, & Masselink, 2014). CCLs are ambassadors for NHCI, helping to link affiliated practices with services and resources provided and also providing an additional helping hand in hallways and infusion areas. CCLs also are patient advocates, identifying resource-based and financial patient needs and linking patients and caregivers with resources best suited to meet their needs. Finally, CCLs empower patients and caregivers by making resources available to them to manage disease and the continuum of care.

## What is next for the NHCI Oncology Patient Navigation Program?

Moving forward, NHCI has three objectives for its patient navigation program:
- Expand metric identification and gathering.
- Revise software systems to meet the needs of the growing program and allow for greater intrasystem navigation.
- Continue expanding and integrating ONNs and CCLs throughout the system.

## Summary and Key Points

A need exists for both nurse and lay navigators within healthcare systems, as both bring tremendous benefit to patients with cancer and their families. In 2005, the National Cancer Institute began studying navigation with the Patient Navigation Research Project. With additional emphasis placed on navigation in NCI's Community Cancer Center Program and the creation of the American College of Surgeons Commission on Cancer patient navigation standard, programs all over the country have started developing their own navigation programs.

Although every navigation program is different, NHCI's program was created with standard steps, providing a blueprint for other programs. Dedicated leadership of the navigation program, along with a systematic design process pulled from a vast array of information and resources, gave the program a strong foundation. This strong foundation and framework (80% of the program), combined with allowance for individualization within the disease site (20%), has contributed to the program's success.

The NHCI program continues to evolve, as it employs continual evaluation, develops assessment tools, and changes based on the needs of patients, caregivers, and the system.
- Careful evaluation of the healthcare system and its current processes—both inpatient and outpatient—is crucial prior to the design of any new navigation program.
- To avoid role confusion and ineffectiveness, it is imperative that ONN core competencies are used and role delineation and scope of practice are determined.

- Careful assessment of how patients with cancer move through a specific healthcare system will allow identification of gaps in care, consequently enabling effective and useful algorithms for navigation.
- Assessment is a cornerstone of nursing practice and the practice of ONNs. Careful, in-depth assessment of the oncology patient allows for a plan to meet patient and caregiver needs and inform other healthcare team members of potential issues.
- Every patient with cancer does not necessarily need or want to be navigated; however, all should be aware of navigation and have access to it.

## Questions

### What is the importance of core competencies in oncology patient navigation?

Core competencies provide the "fundamental knowledge, skills, and expertise required" for navigators to proficiently perform their role (ONS, 2013, p. 7). These competencies can be used for all levels of ONNs—from novice to experienced—as well as for administrators and institutions developing job descriptions, training tools, and materials; evaluating processes; and addressing personal or professional development for ONNs (ONS, 2013).

### Why is patient-centered care as important as evidence-based care?

*Evidence-based practice*, the use of available research and clinical expertise focusing on the best patient outcomes, seems to be at odds with the idea of *patient-centered care*, where patients are "listened to, informed, respected, and involved in their care; and their wishes are honored" (Epstein & Street, 2011, p. 100). The best outcomes need to be defined by what is "meaningful and valuable to the individual patient" (Epstein & Street, 2011, p. 100).

## References

Advisory Board Company. (2011). Maximizing the value of patient navigation: Lessons for optimizing program performance. Retrieved from https://www.advisory.com/research/oncology-roundtable/studies/2011/maximizing-the-value-of-patient-navigation

Blaseg, K. (2009). Patient navigation at Billings Clinic: An NCI Community Cancer Centers Program (NCCCP) pilot site. In *ACCC's cancer care patient navigation: A call to action* (pp. S15–S24). Retrieved from https://www.accc-cancer.org/resources/pdf/PatientNavigation-Guide/s15.pdf

Epstein, R.M., & Street, R.L., Jr. (2011). The values and value of patient-centered care. *Annals of Family Medicine, 9*, 100–103. doi:10.1370/afm.1239

Fillion, L., Cook, S., Veillette, A.-M., Aubin, M., de Serres, M., Rainville, F., … Doll, R. (2012). Professional navigation framework: Elaboration and validation in a Canadian context [Online exclusive]. *Oncology Nursing Forum, 39*, E58–E69. doi:10.1188/12.ONF.E58-E69

Fitch, M. (2008). Supportive care framework. *Canadian Oncology Nursing Journal, 18*, 6–24. Retrieved from http://www.canadianoncologynursingjournal.com/index.php/conj/issue/view/33

Gentry, S.S., & Sellers, J.B. (2014). Navigation considerations when working with patients. In K.D. Blaseg, P. Daugherty, & K.A. Gamblin (Eds.), *Oncology nurse navigation: Delivering patient-centered care across the continuum* (pp. 71–120). Pittsburgh, PA: Oncology Nursing Society.

Mack, N.A., & Shalkowski, L. (2014). How to start and expand a nurse navigation program. In K.D. Blaseg, P. Daugherty, & K.A. Gamblin (Eds.), *Oncology nurse navigation: Delivering patient-centered care across the continuum* (pp. 43–70). Pittsburgh, PA: Oncology Nursing Society.

Oncology Nursing Society. (2013). *Oncology nurse navigator core competencies*. Retrieved from https://www.ons.org/sites/default/files/ONNCompetencies_rev.pdf

Pratt-Chapman, M.L., Willis, L.A., & Masselink, L. (2014). *Core competencies for nonclinically licensed patient navigators*. Washington, DC: The George Washington University Cancer Institute Center for the Advancement of Cancer Survivorship, Navigation and Policy.

Swanson, J.R., Strusowski, P., Mack, N., & Degroot, J. (2012). Growing a navigation program: Using the NCCCP Navigation Assessment Tool. *Oncology Issues, 27*, 36–45. Retrieved from http://www.accc-cancer.org/oncology_issues/articles/JA12/JA12-Growing-a-Navigation-Program.pdf

# Integrating Lay Navigators Within an Existing Nurse Navigator Program

Debbie Bickes, RN, MN, OCN®

Northside Hospital is a community-based hospital system in Atlanta, Georgia, with a comprehensive cancer program, including surgical, medical, and radiation oncology services. Northside also provides comprehensive multidisciplinary support services, including prevention and education, diagnosis, clinical research, genetic counseling, patient navigation, treatment and rehabilitation, individual and group support, survivorship, and palliative care. The hospital system consists of three hospitals that serve metropolitan Atlanta and its surrounding counties. Recent expansion has resulted in an integrated cancer care network with additional locations throughout the state of Georgia. Prior to statewide expansion, Northside's navigation program consisted of several site-specific nurse navigators. Tremendous growth in the volume of patients from the expansion led to an increase in the number of patients with nonclinical barriers to care, especially related to transportation and financial access to care. Barriers related to transportation, finances, and assistance with activities of daily living commonly have been cited as time-consuming to resolve (Fleisher et al., 2012; Hendren et al., 2011; Lin et al., 2008).

## What led to the addition of the lay navigator at Northside?

Northside's participation as an affiliate with the University of Alabama at Birmingham (UAB) Cancer Care Network led to an opportunity to participate in the Health Care Innovation Challenge Awards grant from the Centers for Medicare and Medicaid Services (CMS). The grant allowed for the introduction and incorporation of four lay navigators into the existing Northside nurse navigation team, resulting in converting the Northside navigation model to a blended model of patient navigation.

## What are the benefits of a blended patient navigation model?

A blended patient navigation model using lay and professional navigators has been supported in the literature. Lantz, Keeton, Romano, and DeGroff (2004) described a blended model of navigation in which professional navigators work with patients to serve as clinical guides through their continuum of care, and lay navigators work with patients to ensure that nonclinical issues do not interfere with the ability to continue care. The Center for Health Affairs (2012) stated that relying on highly trained clinical professionals to provide nonclinical services may not be the most efficient use of limited healthcare resources. The Center further stated that lay navigators can carry out important nonclinical tasks while allowing professional navigators to focus their time and attention on the clinical-related functions of their roles. This finding was supported in a study by Koh, Nelson, and Cook (2011). Published studies of lay navigation programs concluded that integration of nonclinical and clinical navigators is needed (McVay, Toney, & Kautz, 2014; Shelton et al., 2011), with one study concluding that the integration of clinical navigation is essential (Fleisher et al., 2012).

## How did Northside plan for the lay navigator role?

The UAB CMS grant structure stipulated that lay navigators report to a nurse program coordinator. The program coordinator is a certified oncology nurse with experience as an oncology nurse navigator (ONN) at Northside and within the hospital's system, oncology support services, and the surrounding community.

A review of the literature at the time of the lay navigator role integration at Northside resulted in the discovery of very few published papers delineating the roles of the clinical and lay navigator. A publication by Canadian Partnership Against Cancer (2012) stressed the importance of clearly defining each navigation role, emphasizing that lay and professional navigation roles are not opposites but rather complement one another by covering distinct tasks and areas of responsibility.

The complementary nature of the two roles was further illustrated in a navigation grid, which provided an overview of professional and lay navigation characteristics and services in seven supportive care domains. This allowed for the comparison of general similarities and differences between the roles (see Figure 2-1). The grid also served as a reference for the delineation of the ONN and lay navigator roles at Northside Hospital, taking into consideration hospital-specific needs, patient population, and UAB CMS grant requirements.

For further delineation of the Northside navigation team members, the title of *lay navigator* was changed to *cancer care liaison* (CCL), with the goal of reducing role confusion for patients and healthcare professionals. The program coordinator collaborated with the oncology patient navigation coordinator to write the CCL job description; delineate the responsibilities, functions, and tasks of the ONN and CCL roles; and set processes, workflow, and courses of action prior to implementing the CCL role. Willis et al. (2013) published a consensus-based patient navigation framework that described, compared, and delineated similarities and differences across three types of patient navigators (see Table 2-1). The similarities and differences in this framework were comparable with the delineation of navigator roles and functions at Northside.

## How were CCLs trained and assessed for competency?

A working knowledge of medical terminology was common among CCLs at the onset of the program. Because a majority did not have experience in an oncology setting, they attended training sessions provided by the UAB grant team. The program coordinator developed and provided additional training specific to Northside (see Figure 2-2). Initial and annual competency assessments also were provided to ensure CCL consistency in knowledge and proficiency in job performance. These competencies were assessed

## Figure 2-1. Navigation Grid

**General Definition of Function**
Navigation is a proactive, intentional process of collaborating with a person and his or her family to provide guidance as they negotiate the maze of treatments, services and potential barriers throughout the cancer journey.

**Vision for Cancer Patient Navigation**
Cancer Patient Navigation is part of an integrated system of cancer service delivery. Navigators work with the patient and family and their interdisciplinary team to assess needs, provide supportive care, answer questions, identify and address any barriers to quality care, and facilitate access to needed resources and services. Navigation aims to improve both coordination in services and continuity throughout cancer care, as well as quality of life for the patient and family throughout the cancer journey.

**Overarching Goal of Navigation Programs**
Navigation programs aim to improve a person's cancer journey by:
• Increasing capacity for knowledge and support
• Increasing capacity to meet identified needs
• Reducing anxiety
• Overcoming barriers and increasing capacity to access clinical and psychosocial services
• Improving coordination among individual services at various points and ensuring continuity across all services

| Role Descriptions | Professional Navigator | Peer/Lay Navigator |
|---|---|---|
| Characteristics | • Is a health professional with specialized knowledge of oncology<br>• Is part of an interprofessional team; provides an effective clinical function<br>• Performs formal, standardized clinical assessment and intervention | • Is a trained peer/lay person, sometimes paid<br>• Is often a person with a cancer experience<br>• Provides person-centered care<br>• Provides general information about cancer journey |

(Continued on next page)

## Figure 2-1. Navigation Grid (Continued)

| Role Descriptions | Professional Navigator | Peer/Lay Navigator |
|---|---|---|
| Characteristics (cont.) | • Provides person-centered care; ensures care team is aware of need for and meaning of a person-centered approach<br>• Creates and follows a care plan at certain points or throughout cancer journey in consultation with team and person/family<br>• Is familiar with and collaborates with peer/lay navigators where applicable<br>• Engages in a proactive, intentional process<br>• Coordinates care and services<br>• Actively monitors care at certain points or throughout cancer journey<br>• Intervenes within scope of practice on patient's and family's behalf<br>• Establishes linkages and coordinates care among agencies and service providers<br>• Provides direct referrals, as desired by patient or family, to other professionals and services<br>• Provides education about disease and related issues and self-care<br>• Provides emotional support during cancer journey | • Focuses on support, empowerment and self-care for patient<br>• Is familiar with and collaborates with professional navigators where applicable<br>• Engages in a proactive, intentional process<br>• Acts in response to concerns identified by patient and family within scope of role<br>• Provides links or facilitates referrals to community agencies and service providers<br>• May facilitate referrals to health care professionals as needed and within scope of role<br>• Provides emotional support and/or shares personal experience within role guidelines<br>• Supports communication with health care providers<br>• May intervene at certain points or throughout the cancer journey<br>• May advocate for patient through health care team within role guidelines<br>• Assists with record-keeping in accordance with patient and/or organizational requirements and privacy legislation |

(Continued on next page)

## Figure 2-1. Navigation Grid *(Continued)*

| Role Descriptions | | Professional Navigator | Peer/Lay Navigator |
|---|---|---|---|
| Characteristics *(cont.)* | | • Works with patient, family and community to facilitate transitions<br>• Provides information, support and guidance in decision-making<br>• Has access to medical records<br>• Maintains record of navigation in accordance with institutional standards and privacy legislation | |
| Services Provided in Seven Supportive Care Domains | 1. Informational | Information and advice about disease, process of treatment, side-effects, services, quality of life, adaptation and changes in ability; instruction in self-management; assistance in decision-making | Information about self-management, tips, services; information about cancer journey process; peer/lay perspective on experience of cancer; support decision-making; encouragement to seek help from professionals and community organizations |
| | 2. Psychological | Comprehensive assessment; professional intervention based on standards of practice; facilitated referral as needed | Identification of concerns, response, validation; peer/lay perspective on experience; offer of hope; encouragement to seek help from professionals and community organizations; referral to resources |

*(Continued on next page)*

**Figure 2-1. Navigation Grid (Continued)**

| Services Provided in Seven Supportive Care Domains (cont.) | | |
| --- | --- | --- |
| 3. Emotional | Comprehensive assessment; professional intervention based on standards of practice; facilitated referral as needed; support in dealing with family's reactions; support for patient and family to express needs to care team; identification of and building on patient's and family's strengths | Identification of concerns, response, validation; peer/lay perspective on experience; normalization of experience; encouragement to seek help from professionals and community organizations |
| 4. Spiritual | Comprehensive assessment; professional intervention based on standards of practice; facilitated referral as needed | Identification of concerns, response, validation; peer/lay perspective on experience; encouragement to seek help from professionals and community organizations |
| 5. Physical | Comprehensive assessment; specific professional interventions and facilitated referral as needed; follow-up on interventions used; consideration of medical history; information about possible symptoms, symptom and pain management; medication changes; decreased fragmentation across care team throughout the continuum of care | Identification of concerns, response, validation; peer/lay perspective on experience; encouragement to seek help from professionals for medical concerns |
| 6. Social | Comprehensive assessment; professional intervention based on standards of practice; facilitated referral as needed; provides broad perspective to care team about specific patient and family situation | Identification of concerns, response, validation; peer/lay perspective on experience; encouragement to seek help from professionals and community organizations |

(Continued on next page)

**Figure 2-1. Navigation Grid (Continued)**

| | | |
|---|---|---|
| Services Provided in Seven Supportive Care Domains (cont.) | 7. Practical | Comprehensive assessment; professional intervention based on standards of practice; facilitated referral as needed | Identification of concerns, response; validate; offer peer/lay perspective on experience; encouragement to seek help from professionals and community organizations; some direct services (e.g., filling out forms, connecting to transportation, translation) |
| Scope of Practice in Key Areas | Assessing needs and existing resources/ strengths | Provides systematic screening/triage and comprehensive clinical assessment for patients and families using standardized, evidence-based tools | Within scope of role, identifies needs and responds to concerns identified by patient and family |
| | Education | Offers standard and personalized medical and psychosocial information and explanation for patient and family, throughout the continuum of care, based on expert knowledge/skill set in oncology | Provides information about patient experience: identifies expected events and related concerns; provides basic health care information |
| | Access | Provides direct referrals to other professionals and services as required following clinical assessment | Encourages help-seeking from professionals; may facilitate referrals to professionals in some cases, according to defined scope of role; provides contacts for practical and support services |

(Continued on next page)

**Figure 2-1. Navigation Grid *(Continued)***

| Scope of Practice in Key Areas *(cont.)* | | |
| --- | --- | --- |
| Support | Provides emotional/psychological support; aids with decision-making based on expert clinical knowledge; focuses on empowerment, building on patient's and family's strengths and resources | Provides emotional support based on extensive peer/lay support training and/or experience; supports patient decision-making; helps to empower the person |
| Coordination | Designs care plan within scope of discipline, participates in interdisciplinary care plan, coordinates care across settings, sets up appointments, explains upcoming appointments/procedures, helps to integrate services; is central point of contact and communication with all health care team members and service providers throughout the continuum of care; is a direct link to tumor board networks; has access to and can share medical records; monitors and evaluates plan of care | Links patient to community resources; encourages help-seeking from professionals; may facilitate referrals to health care professionals as needed and within scope of role |
| Brokering | Actively negotiates for service delivery to clients with the range of professionals and administrators | — |
| Advocacy | Advocates directly for patient with care providers and services, intervenes regarding problems or barriers, advocates for system changes when gaps and inefficiencies are identified | Encourages self-advocacy, empowerment of person |

*(Continued on next page)*

**Figure 2-1. Navigation Grid *(Continued)***

| Scope of Practice in Key Areas *(cont.)* | | |
|---|---|---|
| Documentation | Maintains detailed clinical records, integrates with medical file, monitors care according to professional and institutional standards | Records patient information in some cases, according to defined scope of role and agency expectations |
| System-level change | May identify system barriers (gaps in services, problems with procedures or policies) in the course of daily interactions with patients, and intervene to address/improve them in consultation with interprofessional team and/or administration; may perform patient advocacy and co-ordination across services and professionals, improving care systems | May identify gaps in services, problems with procedures or policies in the course of daily interactions with patients, and communicate concerns to appropriate person in the organization |
| Leadership/ Team building | Provides leadership and influences clinical standard-setting, policy development and change management; promotes and facilitates an interdisciplinary team approach to delivery of care and decision-making; provides leadership in the coordination and implementation of quality improvement activities; facilitates the development and implementation of care pathways | May act as representative on a team, helping to create programs to address identified gaps; offers peer/lay-based leadership and support to other volunteers or participates in mentoring |

*(Continued on next page)*

**Figure 2-1. Navigation Grid (Continued)**

| Skills and training | • Health professional—often a nurse or a social worker<br>• Extensive clinical knowledge of oncology and/or sub-specialty in specific cancer site<br>• Specialized training in navigation process and best practices<br>• Ability to network and coordinate care among all resources, services and professionals<br>• Interpersonal communication and listening skills<br>• Empathy and sensitivity<br>• Knowledge of psychosocial issues, specific needs, possible barriers to care for diverse populations (e.g., cultural, racial, sexual, religious)<br>• Expert in family dynamics<br>• Conflict resolution skills<br>• Awareness of provincial and community cancer agencies, services and resources<br>• Ability to work autonomously<br>• Training in telepractice | • Knowledge of volunteer role and boundaries<br>• Training in navigation process and best practices at peer/lay level<br>• Interpersonal communication and listening skills<br>• Empathy and sensitivity<br>• Ability to maintain client confidentiality and privacy<br>• Knowledge of conflict resolution and incident reporting process<br>• Awareness of limits to knowledge-sharing and when to refer<br>• Knowledge of psychosocial issues, needs, possible barriers to care for diverse populations (e.g., cultural, racial, sexual, religious)<br>• Awareness of provincial and community cancer agencies, services and resources<br>• Professional language translation skills in some cases; ability to access translation services |
| --- | --- | --- |

(Continued on next page)

## Figure 2-1. Navigation Grid *(Continued)*

| | |
|---|---|
| Expected Outcomes | • The cancer experience is improved for the person and family; all are:<br> – Well informed<br> – Prepared with a tailored care plan, with navigator as focal point of contact<br> – Supported and guided<br> – Empowered to make treatment-related decisions<br> – Better equipped to manage anxiety and distress<br>• Barriers to care are identified and addressed; gaps across care path are improved<br>• Disparities are reduced for marginalized groups<br>• Transition points are well managed<br>• The person and family are:<br> – Better informed<br> – Supported and guided<br> – Empowered to make decisions about non-medical issues<br> – Better able to manage anxiety and distress<br> – Empowered to communicate better with health care providers, family and others<br>• Barriers are identified and addressed, within scope of program |
| Possible Modalities | • Face-to-face meetings<br>• Telephone consultation (telemedicine, telepractice)<br>• Online communication (email, chat rooms, online support groups)<br>• Referrals to web-based information (websites, databases)<br>• Referrals to other information sources (resource centres, health libraries, articles, books) |
| Possible Locations | • Clinic/hospital: outpatient or inpatient<br>• Community organization<br>• Home<br>• Online |

*(Continued on next page)*

## Figure 2-1. Navigation Grid *(Continued)*

| | |
|---|---|
| Resource Requirements | • Compensation (for professionals/clinicians; for peer/lay navigators in some cases)<br>• Extensive training curricula, targeted to specific roles and institutional demands<br>• Patient education/information materials<br>• Information about and links to provincial and local resources<br>• Instructors/supervisors<br>• Curriculum developers<br>• Mechanisms to support navigators in work, to debrief and to alleviate emotional stress (e.g., mentoring, professional networks, communities of practice)<br>• Institutional space/office supplies/technical support<br>• Program administration and management<br>• Monitoring and evaluation of programs and individual practice |
| Critical Success Factors | • Leadership<br>• Participation<br>• Problem assessment/problem solving<br>• Organizational structures/processes (e.g., best practice guidelines, accountability framework)<br>• Resource mobilization; referral pathways and links<br>• Communications plan; marketing of program<br>• Right people with the right skillsets<br>• Program management/coordination<br>• Program evaluation mechanisms |

*Note.* From "Guide to Implementing Navigation," by Cancer Journey Action Group, Canadian Partnership Against Cancer, 2010. Retrieved from https://content.cancerview.ca/download/cv/treatment_and_support/supportive_care/documents/guideimplementnavpdf?attachment=0. Copyright 2010 by Cancer Journey Action Group, Canadian Partnership Against Cancer. Reprinted with permission.

---

**Figure 2-2. Northside Hospital Cancer Care Liaison Initial Training and Competency Assessment**

**Topics and Skills**
- Oncology nurse navigator and cancer care liaison role delineation
- Age-specific principles of geriatric care
- Documentation
- Clinical trials
- Resource research and selection
- Communication and listening
- Patient empowerment
- Coping with change
- Cultural diversity and sensitivity
- Challenges common to patients with cancer
- Medicare basics
- Health literacy

**Cancer Care Liaison Competency Verification Methods**
- Case study
- Exemplar
- Test
- Quality improvement monitors
- Self- and peer-assessment
- Return demonstration
- Discussion group
- Presentation

*Note.* Based on information from Wright, 2005.

---

and verified by the program coordinator prior to the CCL initiating patient contact. The CCL role was first piloted in one disease site, with remaining disease sites added as CCLs gained experience and confidence.

In 2014, the George Washington University Cancer Institute (GWUCI) published core competencies for non–clinically licensed patient navigators to assist with standardizing the navigation profession (Pratt-Chapman, Willis, & Masselink, 2014, 2015). These competencies included functional domains, with a total of 45 core competency statements (see Figure 2-3).

Members of the Northside navigation team participated in patient navigator focus groups and a national survey conducted by GWUCI to provide input for validating their core competency statements. The published GWUCI core competencies may be used in future training and development for CCLs at Northside.

**Table 2-1. Patient Navigation Framework: Navigator Function Across Domains**

| Domain | Community (Community Health Worker) | Community/Healthcare Institution (Patient Navigator) | Healthcare Institution (Nurse Navigator/ Social Work Navigator) |
|---|---|---|---|
| **Professional Roles and Responsibilities:** The knowledge base and skills needed to perform job-related duties and tasks, including understanding scope of practice, supporting evaluation efforts, and identifying and exercising self-care strategies.<br><br>The following general skills are required:<br>Organizational skills<br>Office skills<br>Interpersonal skills<br>Time management<br>Problem solving<br>Multitasking<br>Critical thinking | General knowledge base on health issues such as cancer, diabetes, obesity, heart disease, stroke, HIV/AIDS, and other chronic diseases. Active documentation in client record. Conduct evaluation focused on community needs assessment and health behaviors. | Knowledge of cancer screening, diagnosis, treatment, and survivorship and related physical, psychological, and social issues. Active documentation of encounter with patient, barriers to care, and resources or referrals to resolve barriers, which may be noted in the client record and/or the medical record. Conduct evaluation focused on barriers to care, health disparities, and quality indicators. | Knowledge and maintenance of knowledge (e.g., license, certification, continuing education) of cancer clinical impacts on patient, caregivers, and families and ability to intervene (e.g., symptom management, assessment of functional status and psychosocial health). Active documentation in medical record. Conduct evaluation focused on clinical outcomes and quality indicators. |

(Continued on next page)

**Table 2-1. Patient Navigation Framework: Navigator Function Across Domains** *(Continued)*

| Domain | Community (Community Health Worker) | Community/Healthcare Institution (Patient Navigator) | Healthcare Institution (Nurse Navigator/ Social Work Navigator) |
|---|---|---|---|
| **Community Resources:** Ongoing identification, coordination, and referral to resources such as individuals, organizations, and services in the community. | Provide referral to evidence-based health promotion programs. Provide assistance accessing health insurance. | Provide assistance with scheduling appointments and facilitate request and follow-up with specialist or supportive care based on clinical referral. Provide assistance accessing health insurance, copay programs, patient assistance programs, and financial assistance. | Focus on clinically oriented resources, such as referrals for second opinions, treatment or testing that may not be offered at the patient's institution, as well as supportive or specialty referrals within or external to the institution (specific to nurse navigators). |
| **Patient Empowerment:** Identifying problems and resources to help patients solve problems and be part of the decision-making process (see Minnesota Community Health Worker Outline) An important facilitator of patient empowerment is development of good patient rapport. | Motivate individual and community to make positive changes in health behaviors. Activate and empower individuals and communities to self-advocate and make healthy decisions. | Assist patient with identifying administrative, structural, social, and practical issues to participate in decision-making and solutions. Empower patients by ensuring they know all their options; identify their preferences and priorities, and assist them to access healthcare services and self-manage their health. | Assist patients in decision-making regarding diagnostic testing and treatment options (specific to nurse navigators). Provide patients with strategies to cope with disease, treatment, and stress (specific to social work navigators). |

*(Continued on next page)*

**Table 2-1. Patient Navigation Framework: Navigator Function Across Domains *(Continued)***

| Domain | Community (Community Health Worker) | Community/Healthcare Institution (Patient Navigator) | Healthcare Institution (Nurse Navigator/ Social Work Navigator) |
|---|---|---|---|
| **Communication:** Ensuring appropriate communication with patient, healthcare and service providers, and community. | Facilitate communication with community about access and utilization of the healthcare system. | Assist patient and provider with communicating expectations, needs, and perspectives. | Provide translation and communication of clinical information. Provide counseling through one-on-one communication and serve as conduit between patient and providers to address emotional and psychosocial needs of patients (specific to social work navigators). |
| **Barriers to Care/Health Disparities:** Identifying and addressing barriers to care and reducing health disparities as defined by age, disability, education, ethnicity, gender, sexual identification, geographic location, income, or race in populations that often bear a greater burden of disease than the general population. | Address barriers to accessing the healthcare system. Focus on reduction of general health disparities. | Address structural, cultural, social, emotional, and administrative barriers to care. Focus on reduction of cancer health disparities in medically underserved patients and timely access to care across the continuum. | Address clinical and service delivery barriers to care. Provision of services to at-risk populations, which may be defined by individual need, high acuity, or high volume at institutional level. |

*(Continued on next page)*

## Table 2-1. Patient Navigation Framework: Navigator Function Across Domains *(Continued)*

| Domain | Community (Community Health Worker) | Community/Healthcare Institution (Patient Navigator) | Healthcare Institution (Nurse Navigator/ Social Work Navigator) |
|---|---|---|---|
| **Education, Prevention, and Health Promotion:** Promoting healthy behaviors and lifestyle, including integrative and wellness approaches. | Provide general health promotion at the individual and community level, including physical activity, healthy eating habits, stress reduction, sunscreen use, tobacco cessation, and reduction of other risky behaviors to reduce risk of cancer and chronic disease. | Educate patients on practical concerns and next steps in regard to what to expect. Identify the educational needs of patients to advocate on their behalf with the care team. Inform patients of the importance and benefit of clinical trials and connect them with additional resources. | Assess educational needs of patient. Identify the educational needs of patients to advocate on their behalf with the care team. Provide clinical education about diagnosis, treatment, side effects, and posttreatment care (specific to nurse navigators). Educate patients and caregivers on their biopsychosocial concerns regarding their diagnosis and treatment (specific to social work navigators). |

*(Continued on next page)*

| Table 2-1. Patient Navigation Framework: Navigator Function Across Domains *(Continued)* | | | |
|---|---|---|---|
| **Domain** | **Community (Community Health Worker)** | **Community/Healthcare Institution (Patient Navigator)** | **Healthcare Institution (Nurse Navigator/ Social Work Navigator)** |
| **Ethics and Professional Conduct:** Understanding scope of practice and professional boundaries, assuring confidentiality, and following legal requirements. Maintaining and adhering to the professional standards. Bringing accountability, responsibility, and trust to the individuals the profession services. | Abide by state-defined scope of practice. | Understand difference in scope of practice between licensed professionals and non-licensed professionals. | Abide by the ethical principles in the profession's scope of practice and code of conduct according to licensure. |
| **Cultural Competency:** Healthcare services that recognize, respect, and respond to cultural and social differences within the context of beliefs, practices, behaviors, and needs of diverse community and/or population served. | Act as community/cultural liaison and mediator between community and healthcare system using culturally appropriate education materials. | Provide navigation service in a culturally competent manner (e.g., National Culturally and Linguistically Appropriate Services [CLAS] Standards in Health and Health Care). | Provide clinical care and education materials in culturally competent manner. |

*(Continued on next page)*

## Table 2-1. Patient Navigation Framework: Navigator Function Across Domains (Continued)

| Domain | Community (Community Health Worker) | Community/Healthcare Institution (Patient Navigator) | Healthcare Institution (Nurse Navigator/ Social Work Navigator) |
| --- | --- | --- | --- |
| **Outreach:** Providing health-care education to individuals and communities that address health disparities. | Work with the community to identify education needs and opportunities. | Educate on cancer-related topics to reduce fears and barriers related to cancer screening. Effectively link patients referred from the community to resources that can improve care coordination and timeliness to treatment. | Consult and counsel patients on their unique risks. |
| **Care Coordination:** A method of organizing patient care activities to facilitate the appropriate delivery of healthcare services. | Provide care management, service coordination, and system navigation. | Identify the pathway in the continuum and document the next steps to ensure the patient's optimal outcomes. Identify unmet needs and facilitate cancer care resources to eliminate barriers along the cancer continuum. | Assess and facilitate coordination of psychosocial and medical/clinical care along the care continuum. |

(Continued on next page)

**Table 2-1. Patient Navigation Framework: Navigator Function Across Domains (Continued)**

| Domain | Community (Community Health Worker) | Community/Healthcare Institution (Patient Navigator) | Healthcare Institution (Nurse Navigator/ Social Work Navigator) |
|---|---|---|---|
| **Psychosocial Support Services/Assessment:** Providing and/or connecting patients to resources for psychosocial support services. | Identify resources in the community for emotional and social support. | Administer distress screening and provide assistance with administrative, practical, or social issues identified. | Screen and assess for psychosocial distress. Provide psychosocial support services such as counseling (specific to social work navigators). |
| **Advocacy:** Advocating on behalf of patient within the community and healthcare system | Speak up for individual and community needs. | Educate providers on individual preferences of care and needs. | Assure patients' needs and preferences are integrated into treatment and care delivery. |

## How did the addition of the CCL role to the navigation team influence patient care?

The success of the CCL role became apparent shortly after implementation. CCLs were able to focus solely on their patients' practical needs and connect them to resources for resolutions to barriers to care. The UAB CMS grant is specific to the Medicare patient population. Focusing on this specific population has led to an increase in Medicare-specific knowledge, resources, and value for patients and the Northside navigation team. As a result, qualifying Medicare patients have been linked to Medicare savings programs, which have provided assistance with costs.

CCLs have researched, vetted, and created a robust database of resources for the needs of patients with cancer, including financial and transportation assistance for medical care, delivered meals, access to support groups, and free lawn care and housecleaning for patients undergoing chemotherapy. These resources often have assisted patients with activities of daily living, enhancing their ability to live independently during and after cancer treatment.

Resources have been identified and linked to patients according to specific patient-centered needs. For example, a patient experiencing hearing loss was linked to a resource that provided financial assistance for hearing aids. As a result of CCL intervention, the patient was able to hear for the first time in seven years. CCL knowledge of local and national resources and their ability to make additional contacts has resulted in highly successful patient interactions.

CCLs sometimes have served as the actual resource resolution for barriers to care. Some patients have admitted to a trusting CCL that they did not set or attend follow-up appointments in the past because they had grown weary of attending recurrent healthcare visits. The ability to express this frustration to a trusting CCL has contributed to patients following through on attending future appointments.

## How has the CCL role affected ONNs at Northside Hospital?

A CCL's sole focus is on the practical needs of patients. This extra layer of patient support has allowed ONNs to focus their

> ## Figure 2-3. Core Competencies for Non–Clinically Licensed Patient Navigators
>
> **Domain 1: Patient Care**
> Facilitate patient-centered care that is compassionate, appropriate and effective for the treatment of cancer and the promotion of health
>
> 1.1 Assist patients in accessing cancer care and navigating health care systems. Assess barriers to care and engage patients and families in creating potential solutions to financial, practical and social challenges.
> 1.2 Identify appropriate and credible resources responsive to patient needs (practical, social, physical, emotional, spiritual) taking into consideration reading level, health literacy, culture, language and amount of information desired. For physical concerns, emotional needs or clinical information, refer to licensed clinicians.
> 1.3 Educate patients and caregivers on the multi-disciplinary nature of cancer treatment, the roles of team members and what to expect from the health care system. Provide patients and caregivers evidence-based information and refer to clinical staff to answer questions about clinical information, treatment choices and potential outcomes.
> 1.4 Empower patients to communicate their preferences and priorities for treatment to their health care team; facilitate shared decision making in the patient's health care.
> 1.5 Empower patients to participate in their wellness by providing self-management and health promotion resources and referrals.
> 1.6 Follow up with patients to support adherence to agreed-upon treatment plan through continued non-clinical barrier assessment and referrals to supportive resources in collaboration with the clinical team.
>
> **Domain 2: Knowledge for Practice**
> Demonstrate basic understanding of cancer, health care systems and how patients access care and services across the cancer continuum to support and assist patients.
>
> NOTE: This domain refers to foundational knowledge applied across other domains.
>
> 2.1 Demonstrate basic knowledge of medical and cancer terminology.
> 2.2 Demonstrate familiarity with and know how to access and reference evidence-based information regarding cancer screening, diagnosis, treatment and survivorship.
> 2.3 Demonstrate basic knowledge of cancer, cancer treatment and supportive care options, including risks and benefits of clinical trials and integrative therapies.
> 2.4 Demonstrate basic knowledge of health system operations.
> 2.5 Identify potential physical, psychological, social and spiritual impacts of cancer and its treatment.
>
> *(Continued on next page)*

**Figure 2-3. Core Competencies for Non–Clinically Licensed Patient Navigators** *(Continued)*

2.6 Demonstrate general understanding of health care payment structure, financing, and where to refer patients for answers regarding insurance coverage, and financial assistance.

**Domain 3: Practice-Based Learning and Improvement**
Improve patient navigation process through continual self-evaluation and quality improvement. Promote and advance the profession.

3.1 Contribute to patient navigation program development, implementation and evaluation.
3.2 Use evaluation data (barriers to care, patient encounters, resource provision, population health disparities data and quality indicators) to collaboratively improve navigation process and participate in quality improvement.
3.3 Incorporate feedback on performance to improve daily work.
3.4 Use information technology to maximize efficiency of patient navigator's time.
3.5 Continually identify, analyze and use new knowledge to mitigate barriers to care.
3.6 Maintain comprehensive, timely and legible records capturing ongoing patient barriers, patient interactions, barrier resolution and other evaluation metrics and report data to show value to administrators and funders.
3.7 Promote navigation role, responsibilities and value to patients, providers and the larger community.

**Domain 4: Interpersonal and Communication Skills**
Demonstrate interpersonal and communication skills that result in the effective exchange of information and collaboration with patients, their families and health professionals.

4.1 Assess patient capacity to self-advocate; help patients optimize time with their doctors and treatment team (e.g. prioritize questions, clarify information with treatment team).
4.2 Communicate effectively with patients, families and the public to build trusting relationships across a broad range of socioeconomic and cultural backgrounds.
4.3 Employ active listening and remain solutions-oriented in interactions with patients, families and members of the health care team.
4.4 Encourage active communication between patients/families and health care providers to optimize patient outcomes.
4.5 Communicate effectively with navigator colleagues, health professionals and health related agencies to promote patient navigation services and leverage community resources to assist patients.
4.6 Demonstrate empathy, integrity, honesty and compassion in difficult conversations.

*(Continued on next page)*

---

### Figure 2-3. Core Competencies for Non–Clinically Licensed Patient Navigators *(Continued)*

4.7 Know and support National Standards for Culturally and Linguistically Appropriate Services (CLAS) in Health and Health Care to advance health equity, improve quality and reduce health disparities.

4.8 Apply insight and understanding about emotions and human responses to emotions to create and maintain positive interpersonal interactions.

**Domain 5: Professionalism**
Demonstrate a commitment to carrying out professional responsibilities and an adherence to ethical principles.

5.1 Apply knowledge of the difference in roles between clinically licensed and non-licensed professionals and act within professional boundaries.

5.2 Build trust by being accessible, accurate, supportive and acting within scope of practice.

5.3 Use organization, time management, problem-solving and critical thinking to assist patients efficiently and effectively.

5.4 Demonstrate responsiveness to patient needs within scope of practice and professional boundaries.

5.5 Know and support patient rights.

5.6 Demonstrate sensitivity and responsiveness to a diverse patient population, including but not limited to diversity in gender, age, culture, race, religion, abilities and sexual orientation.

5.7 Demonstrate a commitment to ethical principles pertaining to confidentiality, informed consent, business practices and compliance with relevant laws, policies and regulations (e.g. HIPAA, agency abuse reporting rules, Duty to Warn, safety contracting).

5.8 Perform administrative duties accurately and efficiently.

**Domain 6: Systems-Based Practice**
Demonstrate an awareness of and responsiveness to the larger context and system of health care, as well as the ability to call effectively on other resources in the system to provide optimal health care.

6.1 Support a smooth transition of patients across screening, diagnosis, active treatment, survivorship and/or end-of-life care, working with the patient's clinical care team.

6.2 Advocate for quality patient care and optimal patient care systems.

6.3 Organize and prioritize resources to optimize access to care across the cancer continuum for the most vulnerable patients.

*(Continued on next page)*

---

**Figure 2-3. Core Competencies for Non–Clinically Licensed Patient Navigators *(Continued)***

**Domain 7: Interprofessional Collaboration**
Demonstrate ability to engage in an interprofessional team in a manner that optimizes safe, effective patient- and population-centered care.

7.1 Work with other health professionals to establish and maintain a climate of mutual respect, dignity, diversity, ethical integrity and trust.
7.2 Use knowledge of one's role and the roles of other health professionals to appropriately assess and address the needs of patients and populations served to optimize health and wellness.
7.3 Participate in interprofessional teams to provide patient- and population-centered care that is safe, timely, efficient, effective and equitable.

**Domain 8: Personal and Professional Development**
Demonstrate qualities required to sustain lifelong personal and professional growth.

8.1 Set learning and improvement goals. Identify and perform learning activities that address one's gaps in knowledge, skills, attitudes and abilities.
8.2 Demonstrate healthy coping mechanisms to respond to stress; employ self-care strategies.
8.3 Manage possible and actual conflicts between personal and professional responsibilities.
8.4 Recognize that ambiguity is part of patient care and respond by utilizing appropriate resources in dealing with uncertainty.

*Note.* From "Core Competencies for Non-Clinically Licensed Patient Navigators," by M.L. Pratt-Chapman, L.A. Willis, and L. Masselink, 2014. Retrieved from https://smhs.gwu.edu/gwci/sites/gwci/files/PN%20Competencies%20Report.pdf. Copyright 2014 by George Washington University Cancer Institute Center for the Advancement of Cancer Survivorship, Navigation and Policy. Reprinted with permission.

---

time and efforts on the clinical aspects of patient care. Although CCLs focus on the practical needs of patients, patients occasionally also report physical symptoms. Because of the time and emphasis placed on role delineation, process mapping, and competency assessment and verification processes during their initial training, CCLs understand the importance of instructing patients to report clinical symptoms or issues to their physicians. CCLs are instructed to notify the program coordinator and the site-specific ONN when patients report clinical issues. Coordinating with nurses regarding symptoms or clinical issues has provided additional support to the patient and caregiver and has led to a reduction in emergency department visits. CCLs do not cross role boundaries, as they understand and value the expertise and insight that an experienced ONN provides to the clinical aspects of patient navigation. In turn, ONNs trust that CCLs understand their delineated roles and value their expertise in identifying resources and resolving nonclinical barriers to care.

## How do CCLs assist patients at Northside Hospital?

CCLs enhance care and support nonclinical needs of patients at Northside in a multitude of ways. For example, the Northside navigation team received a referral from the radiation oncology department regarding a patient who had "hitched" a ride to the hospital. The patient had been unhappy with the care that he was receiving from healthcare providers at another facility. The radiation oncology staff member stated that the patient needed assistance with transportation and may have other practical needs. The patient met with physicians and healthcare staff. The CCL met with the patient afterward and identified many practical needs.

Because of the multitude of identified needs, the CCL became the primary navigation contact for the patient. The CCL also connected the patient with the site-specific ONN and the program coordinator for clinical concerns. The CCL was able to assist the patient by researching resources for specific needs; providing forms; coordinating and coaching the patient through applications and processes for medical, prescription, and utility bill assistance; coordinating transportation for multiple medical appointments; locating a grocery resource for healthy food (the patient had type 2 diabetes and lived in a "food desert" area of the city); assisting with organizing paperwork; and other areas. The CCL had 268 separate contacts over 18 months with the patient. Many work hours were spent resolving and preventing further barriers to care, missed appointments, and unnecessary emergency department visits.

## What outcomes has the CCL role brought to the Northside navigation team?

The Northside navigation team was built on a framework of person-centered care. The addition of the CCL role has expanded and enhanced the ability of the team to tailor care to the individual needs of patients. CCLs have added a layer of support to connect with patients after discharge, during and after treatment, and at other key times along the continuum of care. This has allowed the navigation team to determine if a patient has had a change in functional status, such as a decrease in the ability to complete activities of daily living or the development of additional obstacles in care. The blended model of navigation has allowed CCLs to link patients with clinical concerns or issues to the site-specific nurse navigator or the program coordinator.

The CCL role also has provided benefits for Northside's older patient population. Patients who qualify under the UAB CMS grant are aged 65 years or older. This older subset often lives alone or lacks a social support network; has at least one chronic condition in addition to a cancer diagnosis; and has other contributory factors that increase the risk to their physical health, diminish their level of functioning, and increase challenges and obstacles to their care (Blank, 2012; Institute of Medicine, 2008).

Additional support from a nonclinical person frequently has led patients to report issues to the CCL that they would otherwise not share with their physicians for fear of being a bother. Often, these issues have the potential to greatly affect care or treatment outcomes. The increase in the number and variety of resources vetted by CCLs has highlighted resolutions for barriers to care not previously reported by patients to clinical professionals. Over time, healthcare professionals at Northside began to realize the value of CCLs and their ability to resolve nonclinical problems faced by patients.

Integration of the CCL role has highlighted the value of the nonclinical navigator role to the Northside navigation team. Similarly, the nonclinical navigator role has underscored the importance of ONNs as members of the navigation team. ONNs provide input, oncology expertise, clinical judgment, and anticipatory guidance for the trajectory of patient care. Gaps in patient care would exist if the navigation team did not work in synchrony.

## Summary and Key Points

Evaluation of the nonclinical CCL role integration into the Northside nurse navigation team has resulted in several conclusions. First, careful and deliberate role delineation with well-defined boundaries was a critical step prior to introduction and implementation of the CCL role. Next, the provision of adequate time for staff training, development, and a competency assessment was crucial to enhance the confidence levels and abilities of CCLs in their role. Finally, communication, collaboration, flexibility, and amenability to change by navigation team members were essential to the successful integration of the nonclinical CCL role into the existing Northside navigation team.

- Role delineation is a key initial step in introducing the nonclinical lay navigator role.
- Staff training for nonclinical lay navigators is important for personal and professional growth.

## Questions

### What is one benefit of adding a nonclinical lay navigator to an existing nurse navigator team?

Nonclinical lay navigators can carry out important nonclinical tasks. This allows the professional navigators to focus their time and attention on clinical-related functions (Center for Health Affairs, 2012; Koh et al., 2011).

### What barriers to care are cited in the literature as the most time-consuming to resolve?

Transportation barriers, financial barriers, and barriers related to assistance with activities of daily living have been cited in the literature as the most time-consuming to resolve (Fleisher et al., 2012; Hendren et al., 2011; Lin et al., 2008).

## References

Blank, T.O. (2012). Theoretical perspectives from gerontology and lifespan experience. In K.M. Bellizzi & M.A. Gosney (Eds.), *Cancer and aging handbook: Research and practice* (pp. 349–364). Hoboken, NJ: Wiley-Blackwell.

Canadian Partnership Against Cancer. (2012). *Navigation: A guide to implementing best practices in person-centered care.* Retrieved from http://www.cancerview.ca/TreatmentAndSupport/PersonCentredCareToolkit/GuidesAndResourcesForChange

Center for Health Affairs. (2012, December). *Issue Brief: The emerging field of patient navigation: A golden opportunity to improve healthcare.* Retrieved from http://www.chanet.org/TheCenterForHealthAffairs/MediaCenter/Publications/IssueBriefs/12-12_Patient-Navigation.aspx

Fleisher, L., Miller, S.M., Crookes, D., Kandadai, V., Wen, K.-Y., Slamon, R.E., & Chaivous, J. (2012). Implementation of a theory-based, non-clinical patient navigator program to address barriers in an urban cancer center setting. *Journal of Oncology Navigation and Survivorship, 3,* 14–23. Retrieved from https://issuu.com/theoncologynurse/docs/jons_june_2012_web?e=1230438/3125732

Hendren, S., Chin, N., Fisher, S., Winters, P., Griggs, J., Mohile, S., & Fiscella, K. (2011). Patients' barriers to receipt of cancer care, and factors associated with needing more assistance from a patient navigator. *Journal of the National Medical Association, 103,* 701–710. Retrieved from http://www.ncbi.nlm.nih.gov/pmc/articles/PMC3713073/pdf/nihms467528.pdf

Institute of Medicine. (2008). *Cancer care for the whole patient: Meeting psychosocial health needs.* Washington, DC: National Academies Press.

Koh, C., Nelson, J.M., & Cook, P.F. (2011). Evaluation of a patient navigation program. *Clinical Journal of Oncology Nursing, 15,* 41–48. doi:10.1188/11.CJON.41-48

Lantz, P.M., Keeton, K., Romano, L., & DeGroff, A. (2004). Case management in public health screening programs: The experience of the National Breast and Cervical Cancer Early Detection Program. *Journal of Public Health Management and Practice, 10,* 545–555. doi:10.1097/00124784-200411000-00012

Lin, C.J., Schwaderer, K.A., Morgenlander, K.H., Ricci, E.M., Hoffman, L., Martz, E., … Heron, D.E. (2008). Factors associated with patient navigators' time spent on reducing barrier to cancer treatment. *Journal of the National Medical Association, 100,* 1290–1297. doi:10.1016/S0027-9684(15)31507-8

McVay, S., Toney, T., & Kautz, D. (2014). The effect of different types of navigators on patient outcomes. *Journal of Oncology Navigation and Survivorship, 5,* 17–24. Retrieved from http://issuu.com/aonn/docs/jons_april14_web

Pratt-Chapman, M.L., Willis, L.A., & Masselink, L. (2014). *Core competencies for non-clinically licensed patient navigators.* Washington, DC: The George Washington University Cancer Institute Center for the Advancement of Cancer Survivorship, Navigation, and Policy. Retrieved from https://smhs.gwu.edu/gwci/sites/gwci/files/PN%20Competencies%20Report.pdf

Pratt-Chapman, M.L., Willis, L.A., & Masselink, L. (2015). Core competencies for oncology patient navigators. *Journal of Oncology Navigation and Survivorship, 6,* 16–21. Retrieved from http://issuu.com/aonn/docs/jons_april15_digital

Shelton, R.C., Thompson, H.S., Jandorf, L., Varela, A., Oliveri, B., Villagra, C., … Redd, W.H. (2011). Training experiences of lay and professional patient navigators for colorectal cancer screening. *Journal of Cancer Education, 26,* 277–284. doi:10.1007/s13187-010-0185-8

Willis, A., Reed, E., Pratt-Chapman, M., Kapp, H., Hatcher, E., Vaitones, V., … Washington, E.-C. (2013). Development of a framework for patient navigation: Delineating roles across navigator types. *Journal of Oncology Navigation and Survivorship, 4,* 20–26.

Wright, D. (2005). *The ultimate guide to competency assessment in health care* (3rd ed.). Minneapolis, MN: Creative Health Care Management, Inc.

# CASE 3
# Increasing the Cancer Workforce With Lay Patient Navigation

Jean B. Sellers, RN, MSN

The University of North Carolina (UNC) Lineberger Comprehensive Cancer Center (LCCC), located in Chapel Hill, is the only public comprehensive cancer center in the state of North Carolina. Its mission includes providing outreach, research, and clinical partnership across the state.

Dare County is located on the eastern shore of North Carolina, extending more than 110 miles from north to south and including the middle part of the Outer Banks and Roanoke Island (Dare County Government, n.d.). Its population is estimated at 35,633 (U.S. Census Bureau, 2015). The region is approximately 240 miles from UNC, with many of its townships remote and difficult to reach (see Figure 3-1). In 2004, cancer was the second leading cause of death in North Carolina and the leading cause of death in Dare County. According to the North Carolina Cancer Registry, cancer mortality rates in Dare County increased by more than 10% between 2000 and 2004. In addition, the county's cancer mortality rate of 219.4 per 1,000 residents was higher than both the state mortality rate of 197.7 and the national mortality rate of 164.3 for 2000–2004 (North Carolina State Center for Health Statistics, 2016). Numerous factors influenced cancer care, including physician referral patterns, affordability, transportation, awareness, and behavioral habits. Geography also was identified by the local health department as a root cause of disparities among this population (Dare County Government, 2010). In 2007, as a response to the growing incidence of cancer in this rural population, a project team was assembled with professionals from UNC LCCC, UNC Health Care, and Dare County. This team identified and recognized the needs and gaps in healthcare services for patients with cancer in this rural county.

## Figure 3-1. Map of Dare County, North Carolina

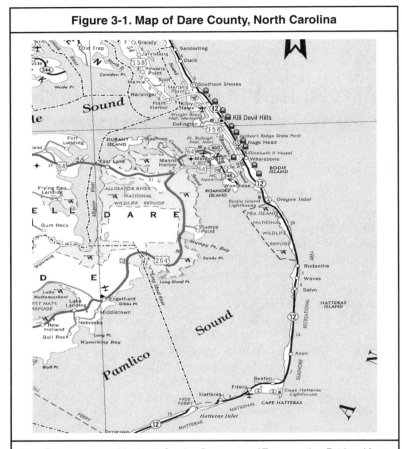

*Note.* Figure courtesy of the North Carolina Department of Transportation. Retrieved from https://xfer.services.ncdot.gov/imgdot/DOTStateTravelMap/dare.jpg. Used with permission.

A number of clinical, education, research, and survivorship goals also were identified (Baer, 2007).

## How was this initiative started?

Face-to-face and telephone interviews with representatives from local hospitals, the local oncologist, physician practices, surgical practices, community support groups, and the Dare County Department of Public Health were used to assess the availability of cancer services in Dare County. The report revealed access to care, affordability, awareness, and behavioral issues as factors that most influenced the cancer care that residents received. As a result of these findings, UNC LCCC and the Dare County Department of Public Health proposed to enhance cancer care in Dare County with the development of a patient navigation model using RNs. This model would include a system of training lay patient advocates to help promote screening and prevention activities while also identifying appropriate methods for accessing the healthcare system. It was envisioned that UNC LCCC would employ and supervise the personnel associated with this project. Initially, personnel included two nurse navigators and an administrative assistant. The nurse navigators would be trained to provide a more sophisticated level of patient assistance to obtain the most appropriate caregivers in specific cases (Campbell, Craig, Eggert, & Bailey-Dorton, 2010). Both groups agreed that the lay navigation model would be incorporated at a later time. Important to the development of this model was an on-site medical director with principal responsibilities for overseeing the training and support of the navigators, identifying new areas of program growth, and coordinating programs with other medical providers in the Outer Banks community. The UNC Outreach Program opened its doors June 2008.

A town hall meeting was called by the Dare County Department of Public Health to bring awareness to the newly developed nurse navigation program designed to assist community members facing a cancer diagnosis. More than 40 people attended the meeting. The Dare County medical oncologist and representatives of the county's health department, government, and local hospital, as well as UNC leadership and UNC nurse navigators, introduced the concept of patient navigation and its importance to the community. Harold Freeman's model was used as an example of how breast cancer outcomes were improved with the integration of patient navigation (Freeman & Rodriguez, 2011). Nurse navigators would address barriers to care, including fear, financial concerns, education, transportation, social isolation, psychosocial concerns, and lack of child or older adult care (Schwaderer & Itano, 2007). Unlike other models, this model would use RNs integrated within the community and not embedded within a practice or cancer center. The program's goals would be to identify and reduce barriers to care and eliminate redundancies in care, reduce the potential for miscommunication among providers, and lessen risk exposure of liability to the navigator. For example, if poorly controlled symptoms are identified, individuals would be referred to their oncology or primary care provider.

At the completion of the presentation, the goals of the program were shared, allowing residents to understand that nurse navigators would help accomplish the following:

- Overcome health system barriers and help facilitate access to care
- Provide information about screening and cancer prevention services available in the community
- Address barriers to care that often accompany a cancer diagnosis
- Link patients to community resources to reduce barriers to care
- Provide psychosocial and emotional support to patients and caregivers

As the nurse navigators concluded their presentation, an older gentleman raised his hand and stood up. He shared that his 32-year-old daughter had died several years prior from cancer and that he did not care much for UNC. The room went quiet. The man continued to say that, in the past 15 years, he had watched UNC and other academic centers bring grant programs in and out of Dare County. Many of these programs presented the promise of providing additional patient support and resources. However, when the funding stopped, the programs often left the county. He continued by saying, "Our people are suffering and dying and we need help. Please do not let this program be like all of the others."

A hush fell over the room. Other members of the community voiced suspicions of a hidden motive for this project and expressed concern that their community eventually would be forgotten or abandoned.

What was most compelling was that these individuals were not interested in the degrees or educational level of presenters. They needed to determine if this group could be true to their word. Did they have character traits that would go beyond persuading people?

## How did the nurse navigators respond to these concerns?

Building trust within any community requires an open and honest approach to communication. In the past, failure to set and communicate realistic expectations for new programs, anticipated outcomes, and duration of support had created mistrust and disappointment within the Dare County community. The nurse navigators quickly acknowledged that what the individuals had stated was true; however, they reassured the group that the program would be integrated into the community at the completion of the funding. The hope was that programmatic costs would be absorbed by the local healthcare organization. It also was noted that a strong partnership had been forged with all community stakeholders, including the county health department, county commissioners, local hospital, and UNC LCCC.

This was a team that had passion, commitment, and heart to improve cancer care and support in the community.

## What was the rationale and design for the proposed nurse-led navigation model?

Professional and experienced oncology nurses understand the importance of collaborative relationships with community partners and have the skills to develop these relationships. Nurse navigator knowledge of current screening and treatment guidelines and awareness of available and reliable community resources is imperative. Nurse navigators understand and can advocate for appropriate symptom and side effect prevention and management, secure financial aid, teach coping and self-management skills, translate dense medical terminology, and promote adherence strategies to medication, treatment, and follow-up protocols. The decision to create a nurse-led navigation model in Dare County was based on these factors.

Selected nurse navigators for Dare County were neither disease specific nor focused on particular socioeconomic groups. Rather, with this area being rural and medically underserved, navigators would serve all patients with cancer and develop strong collaborations with the health department, hospital, and local cancer support community organizations within the county. This role was developed to allow the nurse to meet patients and caregivers at any point in the cancer continuum. These meetings could occur in the patient's home, the physician's office, or a different mutually agreed-upon location.

## What were the challenges in having the community accept the role of the nurse navigator?

Initially, the nurse navigators had to overcome many changes in Dare County. Community healthcare providers were skeptical that the navigators would refer their patients to larger academic centers. Local patients and caregivers expressed an overall mistrust with this new model of support; however, word of mouth quickly spread, as the nurses were able to affect their patients in a positive manner. As one patient said,

> When my cancer returned, one of the nurses at the local clinic mentioned that she had heard of the new UNC nurse navigators located in Nags Head . . . and gave me the phone number. What a blessing that number would be. With one phone call, the UNC nurse navigators had an appointment for me with one of the top specialists in my type of cancer, and within a week, I was at the UNC LCCC getting treatment. That was the first hurdle. From that point on, the nurse navigator regularly called to encourage me and answer my questions—no matter how silly or trivial I thought they might be. She became the friendly voice of caring . . . a personal advocate, providing warmth, compassion, humor, and humanity. My mind cleared, and I formed a plan of recovery. It was much like unfolding a road map. I knew where I was going and all of the different routes to get there without facing roadblocks of decisions or getting lost in my own mind.

## What factors led to the development of the lay navigation model?

Within a year of the initial launch of the nurse navigation model, many challenges continued and new challenges emerged. The number of patients needing support escalated. The percentage of uninsured adults continued to pose problems. Long travel distances and local geography made it difficult for nurse navigators to reach some townships, especially in isolated areas. Community members expressed role confusion with the program and had difficulty finding community cancer support resources.

On January 27, 2009, a group of concerned citizens met in the home of a community member to generate discussion regarding the need for such a program. Community leaders were in attendance and represented Dare County, UNC LCCC, the local health department, the public school system, various community cancer representatives, survivors of cancer, and members of the faith-based community. All agreed that appropriately trained volunteers had the ability to bring a fresh perspective and additional support to the nurse navigation program. Multiple discussions between UNC leadership and key community stakeholders occurred to identify and plan steps to address these issues. Through these discussions, it was determined that many of the value dimensions provided by nurse navigators could be achieved through a cost-effective navigation model using trained volunteer lay health advisors or navigators. Senior leadership at UNC reviewed the role of the lay health advisor and the various models of the lay patient navigator role (Earp et al., 2002).

By developing a model of collaboration among UNC nurse navigators, UNC Health Care's hospital volunteer program, and the community of Dare County, nonclinical support could be provided by volunteers to patients and caregivers. This ultimately would increase the cancer workforce, providing nonclinical support and increasing the number of served residents. The nurse navigator role was expanded to oversee the lay navigators to ensure that nonclinical support would be provided in a safe manner for both volunteers and patients.

The committee continued to meet, eventually developing the guidelines outlined in Figure 3-2.

## What resources were initially provided by UNC LCCC?

The decision to partner with the UNC volunteer program was based on several factors. For one, incorporating trained volunteers into an existing nurse navigation model would provide the hospital with associated cost savings (Hotchkiss, Fottler, & Unruh, 2009). The partnership also would provide program infrastructure that would allow volunteers to be screened according to the policies of the UNC volunteer program. Volunteers were interviewed by the local volunteer coordinator and nurse navigator. They were then selected and vetted through the UNC volunteer program, ensuring that volunteers passed background checks and were current with immunizations. Volunteers partici-

| Figure 3-2. Lay Navigation Guidelines |
|---|
| • Incorporate current UNC Health Care hospital volunteer framework to ensure appropriate screening of volunteers.<br>• Develop a job description, training agenda, training manual, outcome measures, and community cancer resource list.<br>• Partner with local faith-based communities to function as a bridge between people in need, the community healthcare system, and local resources (Rodriguez et al., 2009).<br>• Initiate countywide volunteer recruitment from current survivors of cancer and retired healthcare staff.<br>• Collaborate with local healthcare providers, community organizations that share similar purposes, local churches, and public schools to promote both models of patient navigation. Examples include Rotary Club, Kiwanis Club, Chamber of Commerce, adult and senior daycare centers, cancer support groups, local churches and public school staff meetings, guest interview spots on local radio stations, and educational articles in local newspapers. Program information would be included in local libraries and as inserts in local church bulletins.<br>• With oversight and training from the nurse navigator, lay navigators would provide nonclinical support, including emotional support, assistance with transportation, preparation of meals, and respite and child care for patients and caregivers. The additional dimension of their role should include community education to promote healthy lifestyles and cancer prevention (Bickell & Paskett, 2013). |

pated in the required hospital orientation and Health Insurance Portability and Accountability Act training. Once volunteers had completed this training, they were then able to participate in separate lay navigation training.

## What steps were considered critical for the success of the program?

Table 3-1 outlines the steps critical to the program.

## What were the training components?

Initially, a training manual and two-hour orientation were developed by the UNC Cancer Network and UNC Volunteer Services to support the development of skills and confidence among

**Table 3-1. Critical Steps in Building the Dare County Lay Navigator Program**

| Task | Rationale |
| --- | --- |
| Recruiting a physician champion | The local oncologist was knowledgeable about local healthcare barriers to care, demographics of the local population served, and its culture. |
| Recruiting community stakeholders to serve in an advisory capacity | Representatives from UNC, the local health department, local hospital, local healthcare providers, local cancer support organizations, community organizations, faith-based communities, and cancer survivors will ensure community buy-in. |
| Scheduling bimonthly meetings with a defined agenda and minutes | Tasks:<br>• Community needs assessment review<br>• Mission and vision<br>• Program name |
| Developing training, role delineation, and core competencies | Defining the training, core competencies, and roles of the lay and nurse navigator were important. The model was developed by the UNC Cancer Network for the nurse navigator to provide oversight to the lay navigator (Dohan & Schrag, 2005; Oncology Nursing Society [ONS], 2013; ONS et al., 2010; Pratt-Chapman et al., 2014). |
| Developing clearly defined policies and procedures | Patients were referred in a variety of ways or may self-refer to the program.<br>An intake/evaluation form was completed by the program assistant and entered into a database, and the nurse navigator was informed. The nurse navigator then would assign the patient to the appropriate lay navigator. (Or, after review, the nurse navigator may direct the referral to the volunteer coordinator of the lay navigators.) |
| Developing outcome measures | These measured the success of the program and identified opportunities for improvement. |
| Scheduling monthly lay navigation education meetings | These meetings ensured ongoing skill and confidence building and provided an opportunity for lay navigators to share experiences. |
| Establishing marketing and community outreach | Targeted presentations were held throughout the community to promote awareness of the program and recruit volunteers. |
| Developing a local cancer resource guide | The Dare County cancer resource guide allowed patient navigators, patients, and caregivers to have access to available support resources. |

lay navigators in providing nonclinical support. The curriculum, based on the National Patient Navigator Training Program, was comprehensive and included topics such as a basic understanding of cancer, the essentials of compassionate communication, patient confidentiality, boundary setting, and understanding barriers to care (Calhoun et al., 2010). The training was led by an oncology nurse, a health education specialist, and the UNC Volunteer Services director. All volunteers were given a training manual and a community cancer guide for Dare County that highlighted resources available to assist patients and caregivers. Ongoing training and educational updates were identified as important in the development of these volunteers, as it was impossible to provide all necessary education in the initial training.

On completion of the training, volunteers would be able to accomplish the following:
- Communicate in a respectful and supportive manner
- Provide emotional support within comfortable boundaries for volunteers and patients
- Identify nonmedical barriers to care
- Connect patients with existing cancer support programs and resources

## What efforts were made to promote awareness of the of the program?

Promotional flyers and press releases were developed and distributed within all local community organizations, including faith-based communities, to recruit volunteers and market the program. UNC nurse navigators provided presentations at the local cancer support group, adult and senior daycare services, Kiwanis Club meetings, cancer foundation meetings, Rotary Club, and staff meetings for the public schools.

The advisory committee selected "Hands of Hope" as the program name to ensure its own identity and that it did not duplicate services. The program's focus would be on complementing existing community resources.

It was important to communicate a clear message for the program. This was a grassroots community initiative that arose out of a collective desire to ensure that no one walks the cancer journey alone. The program was nurtured and supported by many individuals, groups, and organizations that joined together to develop a lifeline of support for patients with cancer in need.

Lay navigators were identified as volunteer members of a patient's own community who had received special training regarding the following:

- The basic understanding of what cancer is and is not
- How to communicate with the patient and family affected by cancer
- The need to maintain confidentiality
- The understanding of available community resources

## When was the first training hosted?

The first training was hosted at the local hospital in November 2009. The room was at full capacity, with more than 40 people participating. Within one year, the local hospital had taken an active role in hiring and funding a volunteer coordinator and assumed responsibility for vetting volunteers through its own volunteer association. The lay navigation program was implemented January 2010. Within the first four months, more than 25 volunteers provided an average of 319 service hours and 50 encounters for nine patients per month. Between 2009 and 2010, 78 volunteer navigators completed training.

## What were the successes of the program?

The program had many success stories in a short time period. Trained lay and nurse navigators worked together to provide nonclinical support and education to community members, patients, and caregivers through increasing awareness of available community resources; providing transportation, child care, respite, pet care, social outings, and meal preparation; and coordinating overnight accommodations for medical appointments. Working with the local health department and county government, a partnership with local hotels and motels was established to ensure that future patients and caregivers living outside of the community would have an affordable place to stay when receiving cancer treatment locally. The interventions used are detailed in Figure 3-3.

---

### Figure 3-3. Types of Interventions

- Refer to financial resources.
- Refer to cancer support resources.
- Assist with transportation.
- Assist with meals and picking up supplies.
- Schedule appointments.
- Arrange lodging accommodations.
- Assist with child care or pet care.
- Provide emotional support.
- Coordinate travel for doctor's appointments.
- Accompany to appointments.
- Provide cancer education and resources.
- Facilitate communication.
- Give respite to the caregiver.
- Assist with yard chores.

---

## What were the lessons learned?

UNC LCCC quickly learned from the challenges of developing a new program more than 200 miles away. Because of the distance, it was readily appreciated that local governance of the program was available for long-term success. During a five-year time frame, the program transitioned from being fully funded by UNC LCCC to being fully funded by the local hospital. Initial contributions and funding were significant in the development and integration of this model. Collaborations between hospitals, local healthcare providers, and nearby communities were essential in generating community support. Examples of these partnerships included health departments, social services, existing community nonprofits, faith-based communities, community care clinics, private providers, and senior centers. The natural partnership with the lay volunteer navigation program at the local hospital level was critical in providing infrastructure for this model. This support also was important to the long-term success of both the nurse navigator and lay navigator programs.

This is an example of how outside groups may be able to initiate a navigation program that can eventually be turned over to the local governance for long-term management and control, thus avoiding the criticism of eliminating programs when grant funding lapses.

## What were the complexities of working with volunteers?

Incorporating trained volunteers into an existing program requires significant time and oversight. Many volunteers did not have a healthcare background but were survivors of cancer and demonstrated a desire to help others facing a cancer diagnosis. Ensuring that they had the skills to be effective and confident was critical. It was imperative to have appropriate written policies that were easy to follow. Expanding the role of the nurse navigator to include supervision of lay navigators ensured clear communication (Oncology Nursing Society, 2010). The roles of the nurse navigator and lay navigator were clearly delineated to avoid confusion among the staff and the community. It also was important to ensure that volunteers understood patient confidentiality and the importance of setting appropriate boundaries. By using the hospital's volunteer infrastructure, the program was able to tap into established training and save cost on background checks, immunizations, and other requirements, allowing the development of a model that would save costs and generate positive patient and volunteer feedback. The volunteers were found to be self-motivated and able to provide the additional nonclinical support needed to benefit the local cancer community.

## Summary and Key Points

The navigation program in Dare County originated as part of the UNC Cancer Network and followed the initial work of UNC nurse navigators. The program was the result of a community's belief that no one should face cancer alone.

- The long-term success of a program like this requires ongoing local management and supervision, funding, and early inclusion of local healthcare providers and facilities (e.g., health departments, hospitals).
- Using professional and lay patient navigators is effective in supporting patients with cancer and their caregivers.
- This lay navigator program demonstrated that nonclinical support can be provided to improve the cancer experience and reach underserved patients.

• As models of patient navigation evolve, additional evidence to support models of care must be identified.

## Questions

### What is most important in the development of a specific geographic navigation program?

Having an understanding of the needs of the individual community and its available resources is critical prior to implementing outreach models of patient navigation.

### Who is qualified to initiate and direct a regional program with lay navigators?

Certified oncology nurses are in a position to oversee trained nonprofessional volunteers to provide nonclinical support for patients and caregivers.

## References

Baer, A. (2007, December 5). Cancer hospital aims to improve local care. *Outer Banks Sentinel.* Retrieved from http://www.obsentinel.com/features/cancer-hospital -aims-to-improve-local-care/article_4eb753d2-7740-5679-a939-ef061b63a39c.html

Bickell, N.A., & Paskett, E.D. (2013). Reducing inequalities in cancer outcomes: What works? *American Society of Clinical Oncology Educational Book, 2013,* e250– e254. doi:10.1200/EdBook_AM.2013.33.e250

Calhoun, E.A., Whitley, E.M., Esparza, A., Ness, E., Greene, A., Garcia, R., & Valverde, P.A. (2010). A national patient navigator training program. *Health Promotion Practice, 11,* 205–215. doi:10.1177/1524839908323521

Campbell, C., Craig, J., Eggert, J., & Bailey-Dorton, C. (2010). Implementing and measuring the impact of patient navigation at a comprehensive community cancer center. *Oncology Nursing Forum, 27,* 61–68. doi:10.1188/10.ONF.61-68

Dare County Government. (n.d.). History. Retrieved from http://www.darenc.com/ general/history.asp

Dare County Government. (2010). 2010 community health profile. Retrieved from http://www.darenc.com/health/docs/CommHlthPrfle.pdf

Dohan, D., & Schrag, D. (2005). Using navigators to improve care of underserved patients: Current practices and approaches. *Cancer, 104,* 848–855. doi:10.1002/cncr.21214

Earp, J.A., Eng, E., O'Malley, M.S., Altpeter, M., Rauscher, G., Mayne, L., ... Qaqish, B. (2002). Increasing use of mammography among older, rural African American women: Results from a community trial. *American Journal of Public Health, 92,* 646– 654. doi:10.2105/AJPH.92.4.646

Freeman, H.P., & Rodriguez, R.L. (2011). History and principles of patient navigation. *Cancer, 117*(Suppl. 15), 3537–3540. doi:10.1002/cncr.26262

Hotchkiss, R.B., Fottler, M.D., & Unruh, L. (2009). Valuing volunteers: The impact of volunteerism on hospital performance. *Health Care Management Review, 24,* 119–128. doi:10.1097/HMR.0b013e31819e919a

North Carolina State Center for Health Statistics. (2016). Statistics and reports: Cancer. Retrieved from http://www.schs.state.nc.us/data/cancer.cfm

Oncology Nursing Society, Association of Oncology Social Work, & National Association of Social Workers. (2010). *Oncology Nursing Society, the Association of Oncology Social Work, and the National Association of Social Workers joint position statement on the role of oncology nursing and oncology social work in patient navigation.* Retrieved from https://www.ons.org/sites/default/files/Role%20of%20Social%20Worker.pdf

Oncology Nursing Society. (2013). *Oncology nurse navigator core competencies.* Retrieved from https://www.ons.org/sites/default/files/ONNCompetencies_rev.pdf

Pratt-Chapman, M.L., Willis, L.A., & Masselink, L. (2014). *Core competencies for non-clinically licensed patient navigators.* Washington, DC: The George Washington University Cancer Institute Center for the Advancement of Cancer Survivorship, Navigation, and Policy. Retrieved from https://smhs.gwu.edu/gwci/sites/gwci/files/PN%20Competencies%20Report.pdf

Rodriguez, E.M., Bowie, J.V., Frattaroli, S., & Gielen, A. (2009). A qualitative exploration of the community partner experience in a faith-based breast cancer educational intervention. *Health Education Research, 24,* 760–771. doi:10.1093/her/cyp010

Schwaderer, K.A., & Itano, J.K. (2007). Bridging the healthcare divide with patient navigation: Development of a research program to address disparities. *Clinical Journal of Oncology Nursing, 11,* 633–639. doi:10.1188/07.CJON.633-639

Sheldon, L.K. (2005). Communication in oncology care: The effectiveness of skills training workshops for healthcare providers. *Clinical Journal of Oncology Nursing, 9,* 305–312. doi:10.1188/05.CJON.305-312

U.S. Census Bureau. (2015). Quickfacts: Dare County, North Carolina. Retrieved from http://www.census.gov/quickfacts/table/PST045215/37055

# CASE 4
# Ethics: Supporting the Family Journey

Alice S. Kerber, MN, APRN, ACNS-BC, AOCN®, AGN-BC

A.T. is a 29-year-old woman with a strong family history of breast and ovarian cancers. A.T. first contacts her oncology nurse navigator (ONN) at a community center free clinic. A.T.'s ONN, who also is a genetic nurse specialist employed in the clinic as part of grant funding, was introduced to A.T. by her nurse practitioner (NP), who thought A.T. could benefit from counseling and possibly some testing to guide surveillance and management. The center clinic staff was working on a project to identify women at high risk for breast and ovarian cancer who might not otherwise have genetic counseling or testing. A.T. has no health insurance to cover genetic counseling or testing, but she does have a strong family history. She comes to the clinic with a worrisome breast finding and a history of benign ovarian fibroids.

## What questions should the ONN ask the patient to adequately assess family history?

When assessing family history, the ONN should ask questions designed to assess both the probability of cancer in the future and the potential benefits of counseling or testing. Questions concerning family history should be designed to initiate conversation about health issues in the family. Such conversations can help identify conditions and detect patterns of behavior, environment, or genetics that may increase or decrease cancer risk; provide opportunities to reinforce healthy behaviors; and educate about cancer prevention and surveillance in a high-risk family (American Nurses Association [ANA] & International Society of Nurses in Genetics [ISONG], 2016). Helpful information to gather includes the following:

- Family history (three generations of both the maternal and paternal sides of the family)
  - Major health conditions
  - Age at which diseases developed
  - Age and cause of death
  - Ethnic backgrounds
  - Pregnancy problems
  - General lifestyle of family
- Information about the patient's first-, second-, and third-degree relatives on both sides of the family
  - A first-degree relative is a close blood relative and includes parents, full siblings, and children.
  - A second-degree relative is a blood relative and includes grandparents, grandchildren, aunts, uncles, nephews, nieces, and half-siblings.
  - A third-degree relative is a blood relative and includes first cousins, great-grandparents, and great-grandchildren.

A.T.'s mother was diagnosed with stage II estrogen receptor (ER)/progesterone receptor (PR)-negative, HER2-positive breast cancer and Paget disease of the right breast at age 39. She had a right breast mastectomy followed by chemotherapy and radiation. After trastuzumab became available, she received it for one year. Because of an abnormal mammogram of the left breast, A.T.'s mother underwent a second mastectomy and transverse rectus abdominis flap surgery at age 51. She had genetic testing with the second diagnosis, and no pathogenic mutation was found in *BRCA1* and *BRCA2* sequencing.

A.T.'s maternal grandfather, at age 89, also was diagnosed with cancer of his right breast. He had surgery for his ER/PR-positive, HER2-negative cancer and took tamoxifen until his death (due to comorbidities) at age 91. He received genetic testing because of the rarity of male breast cancer and was found to have a *BRCA2* mutation.

A.T.'s mother underwent additional testing of the *BRCA1* and *BRCA2* genes for large rearrangement and deletion and duplication. No pathogenic mutation was identified; however, because the pathogenic mutation status identified the family as one with hereditary breast and ovarian cancer syndrome (HBOC), the family is at higher risk for certain HBOC-related cancers. In this situation, heightened surveillance is recommended by the National Comprehensive Cancer Network® (NCCN®); therefore, additional close relatives were tested (NCCN, 2016).

A.T.'s maternal grandfather's two sisters were tested and found to carry the same pathogenic mutation in the *BRCA2* gene. One had been diagnosed with breast cancer at age 80 (and declined treatment due to comorbidities), and the other had been diagnosed with pancreatic cancer at age 84. Both are now deceased, and neither have living children or grandchildren. No information exists concerning any other cancer diagnoses.

A.T.'s two maternal aunts also were tested for the known mutation. One tested negative and continues with routine surveillance, while the other tested positive for the mutation and underwent an elective salpingo-oophorectomy and bilateral mastectomy.

## What are some red flags for hereditary cancers?

When evaluating patients for hereditary cancers, clinicians should red flag the characteristics that may help identify those who could benefit from a genetic counseling referral for additional risk assessment and possible testing (NCCN, 2016). Such red flags may include the following:

- Earlier age at onset of cancer than expected
- Bilateral or multiple primary cancers in the same individual
- Multiple family members affected
- Cancer in a less-often-affected sex
- Rare cancers in absence of known risk factors
- Ethnic predisposition (e.g., Ashkenazi Jewish, Icelandic, Native American)
- Known pathogenic mutation in the family

## What is the role of the ONN in hereditary cancer?

The ONN must stay knowledgeable of the expanding influence of cancer genetics on patients and families. Educating patients and families about hereditary cancer risk and guiding them to appropriate genetics professionals will become more important as the field expands (ANA & ISONG, 2016; Kirk, Calzone, Arimori, & Tonkin,

2011). Responsibilities of the ONN concerning hereditary education may include the following:

• Assess personal and family history for increased genetic risk.
• Educate clients and families about basic genetics.
• Initiate referrals to credentialed genetics professionals for counseling.
• Personalize surveillance and management with genetic information.
• Evaluate the holistic influence of the genetic condition, therapeutics, and testing on the client and their family.
• Expand professional knowledge and expertise through continuing education in genetics and genomics.

## What is A.T.'s entry into the navigation process?

A.T.'s mother is familiar with the community center because she had previously donated tickets for a fund-raising event. A.T. is 29 years old, no longer eligible for healthcare coverage under her mother's plan, has no health insurance despite working two jobs, is living in and contributing to her mother's household, and is raising two children as a single mother. When A.T. had a worrisome breast finding, her mother encouraged her to go to the community center, which offered low- or no-cost health care.

On her initial visit, A.T. is seen by the NP at the clinic for a physical examination. While the examination is taking place, the ONN meets with A.T.'s mother, collects family history, and confirms that A.T. meets the criteria for testing. The breast finding is confirmed, and A.T. is scheduled for a mammogram and ultrasound in the upcoming weeks.

## Does A.T. meet the criteria for financial support for testing?

Affected (confirmed diagnosis of cancer) and unaffected (no known diagnosis of cancer) individuals may be eligible for financial support or compassionate pricing based on specific medical and financial criteria (Assistant Secretary for Planning and Evaluation, 2016; Myriad Genetics Laboratories, n.d.).

The clinic is able to obtain testing for A.T. while she is unaffected and uninsured because she meets financial and medical criteria. The clinic provides documentation of the known mutation as well as A.T.'s proof of income status based on her previous year tax returns and her attestation to income level and insurance status.

## What ethical considerations should the ONN consider when evaluating A.T.?

When an ONN discusses family history and possible genetic relationships, ethical issues must be considered (Monsen, 2009). Ethics play an important role in nurse navigation. Specific principles, such as autonomy (right to self-determination, informed consent), veracity (right to be told the truth in a balanced presentation), justice (equity), fidelity (right to confidentiality, advocacy), beneficence (do the right thing), and nonmaleficence (do no harm), are of utmost importance. Some important questions that the ONN should consider in A.T.'s case include the following:

- Does A.T. need testing?
- Will results change her care?
- Could other family members be helped by this information?
- How much does it cost?
- Does she want testing?
- What are the protections for confidentiality?

## What tests and counseling should A.T. receive?

A.T. receives genetic counseling and pretest education. A.T. has several conversations with her ONN. The process moves quickly, and she confirms that she definitely wants testing. Results of testing should help guide both her surveillance schema and treatment planning.

Because her mother does not have the known familial mutation, A.T. is to be tested first for the known familial mutation and, if negative, have reflex testing to include a panel of 25 genes associated with hereditary cancers. The ONN obtains informed consent.

A.T. tests negative for the known mutation, but with her age at diagnosis, her physician supports and requests additional panel testing. This testing identifies a *BRCA2* variant of uncertain significance

(VUS). Because the VUS is not actionable, A.T.'s treatment plan does not change; however, she will be monitored for additional cancers based on her personal and family history.

## What ethical issues are specific to A.T.?

Working with A.T., the ONN is able to provide accurate, understandable, and usable information. The navigator also is able to place the information in the context of A.T.'s diagnosis and her family. It is decided that A.T.'s siblings and children only will be tested at the appropriate time if A.T.'s VUS is reclassified as pathogenic. The ONN provides access to care despite A.T.'s insurance status. To honor A.T.'s privacy, the ONN also advocates for her choices about who to include in the information and the timing and type of surgery (Monsen, 2009).

## How can personalized management techniques be used with A.T.?

Personalized management is used for patients to identify individual risks as well as opportunities to promote health and appropriate management. The ONN is able to offer a diagnosis and management plan personalized for A.T. With a known familial mutation, A.T. is at an increased risk for many different types of cancers, including breast, ovarian, melanoma, and pancreatic. In A.T., a *BRCA2* VUS is discovered, which provides insufficient data for guidance in management modification. She remains at a higher risk for additional cancers because of her family history. A.T. will need further monitoring in case of reclassification of the VUS, which could influence continuing management of her known cancer and the potential for other cancers (NCCN, 2016).

## Summary and Key Points

With her genetic testing, A.T. also received a breast biopsy, revealing ductal carcinoma in situ. Her genetic test results were uninformative and her siblings did not proceed with testing. Because of her family history, A.T. opted for a double mastectomy with reconstruction. A.T. also plans on a bilateral oophorectomy in the future because of her history of benign but painful ovarian tumors.

- The first step to screening, preventing, and managing hereditary cancer syndromes is recognition.
- Increased surveillance or interventions may identify cancers early or reduce their risks.
- Ethical issues must be considered and addressed in every situation.
- Genetic counseling and risk assessment do not always lead to genetic testing, but lack of knowledge of when to refer, questions about access, or uncertainty regarding insurance coverage should not be major determinants to decision making, as resources are available for guidance and support to the uninformed, uninsured, and underinsured.
- The ONN is vital in providing guidance and advocacy, especially to the underserved or those unsure of the steps in their unique cancer journeys.

## Questions

### What type of individual might benefit from genetic testing?

An example of an individual who might benefit from genetic testing fits the following profile: J.H. is a 25-year-old African American unaffected woman with a history of several family members with breast cancer diagnosed before age 50. A known pathogenic mutation exists in the family.

### What is the principle of fidelity in the ethical sense?

From the client perspective, *fidelity* is the right to confidentiality and the expectation that care will be provided. From the provider perspective, fidelity is respect for personhood and the duty to keep promises (ANA, n.d.).

## References

American Nurses Association. (n.d.). Short definitions of ethical principles and theories: Familiar words, what do they mean? Retrieved from http://www.nursingworld.org/MainMenuCategories/EthicsStandards/Resources/Ethics-Definitions.pdf

American Nurses Association & International Society of Nurses in Genetics. (2016). *Genetics/genomics nursing: Scope and standards of practice* (2nd ed.). Silver Spring, MD: Nursesbook.org.

Assistant Secretary for Planning and Evaluation. (2016). Poverty guidelines. Retrieved from https://aspe.hhs.gov/poverty-guidelines

Kirk, M., Calzone, K., Arimori, N., & Tonkin, E. (2011). Genetics-genomics competencies and nursing regulation. *Journal of Nursing Scholarship, 43,* 107–116. doi:10.1111/j.1547-5069.2011.01388.x

Monsen, R.B. (2009). *Genetics and ethics in health care: New questions in the age of genomic health.* Bethesda, MD: American Nurses Association.

Myriad Genetics Laboratories. (n.d.). Financial assistance program. Retrieved from https://www.myriad.com/myriad-cares-2/financial-assistance-program

National Comprehensive Cancer Network. (2016). *NCCN Clinical Practice Guidelines in Oncology (NCCN Guidelines®): Genetic/familial high-risk assessment: Breast and ovarian* [v.2.2016]. Retrieved from https://www.nccn.org/professionals/physician_gls/pdf/genetics_screening.pdf

# Breast Cancer in an Older Adult Patient

Sharon Gentry, RN, MSN, AOCN®, CBCN®

O.W. is a 70-year-old woman undergoing her annual mammogram at a community imaging center. She feels compelled to participate in annual screenings because her mother had ovarian cancer at age 45, her sister had uterine cancer at age 35, and her maternal grandmother had colon cancer at age 65; all are deceased. The mammogram shows entirely fatty-replaced breasts, except for a left lower inner quadrant asymmetry in the right breast that measures 6 mm on a follow-up ultrasound. A core biopsy reveals a grade 2 invasive ductal carcinoma with luminal-like features of estrogen receptor, progesterone receptor, and HER2 positivity and a Ki-67 of 20% (Boa & Davidson, 2008).

## What is the role of the nurse navigator in breast cancer?

A breast oncology nurse navigator (ONN) can perform patient-centered education on breast cancer type and possible treatment options using an inclusive pathology report. The ONN also can be available during the disease trajectory to proactively guide the patient with additional education and support (Pedersen & Hack, 2010). Contact with a nurse navigator at diagnosis has shown to increase downstream revenue to the healthcare system by retaining patients in the system (Desimini et al., 2011).

O.W. meets with the radiologist and ONN to receive her diagnosis. The ONN follows up on the fluorescence in situ hybridization (FISH) testing from the prognostic panel prior to O.W.'s visit to see if the tumor cells are positive or have extra copies of the *HER2* gene. This would qualify O.W. for a neoadjuvant chemotherapy discussion.

O.W. is FISH negative, so the ONN's next step (per her algorithm) is to arrange a surgeon and radiation oncology visit (see Figure 5-1). Previously at this accredited community cancer center, patients with early-stage disease provided feedback that seeing a medical oncologist prior to surgery was not beneficial. In this case, it would have been an additional co-pay for an older woman living on a fixed income.

## How can the ONN help this patient?

The ONN reviews physical and social elements for patient-centered care. O.W. comes from a rural community that offers breast diagnostic services but no treatment. Her travel time commuting to the cancer center is an hour and a half to two hours round-trip. The ONN notices that O.W. came alone for her results and discovers that her husband is a chronic diabetic with cardiac issues. "He never seems to understand and be compliant with his own health issues," O.W. says.

The couple is living on a fixed income, and all extra money goes to his medical care. She has a part-time job at a local bookstore for "a little extra on the side." Their son died when he was in his 40s due to complications from diabetes mellitus and a deep vein thrombosis.

The couple's 45-year-old daughter lives out of state. "She only is interested in her career and does not desire to visit this area often," says O.W.

O.W. experienced menorrhagia when she was in her mid-40s from uterine fibroids and had a total abdominal hysterectomy and bilateral oophorectomy. She has never taken birth control or hormone replacement therapy. O.W. does not smoke or drink and walks (usually outside) every other day. Her other medical concerns are hypertension controlled with current medication; osteoarthritis, which she grades as a 2 on a 0–10 pain scale on days when she takes over-the-counter medication; and depression. She adamantly states she does not and will not take antidepressants.

At the initial meeting, the ONN identifies some concerns (e.g., transportation, distance for treatment, financial, social, depression, genetics) and strengths (e.g., exercise, independence, no major physical concerns or comorbidities) (see Figure 5-2).

# Figure 5-1. Breast Nurse Navigator Algorithm

| Invasive Cancer* (Goal: All Appointments within 8 Business Days of Diagnosis) | DCIS* | High Risk* (ADH, ALH, LCIS) |
|---|---|---|
| Diagnosis by Image-Guided Core Biopsy | Diagnosis by Image-Guided Core Biopsy | Diagnosis by Image-Guided Core Biopsy |
| Pt to NH Breast Center/KMC for Pathology Result/Navigator Consult *all patients referred from outside sources should be offered Navigation services pre-operatively by surgeon* | Pt to NH Breast Center/KMC for Pathology Result/ Navigator Consult *all patients referred from outside sources should be offered Navigation services pre-operatively by surgeon* | *Pt to NH Breast Center/KMC for Pathology Result/Navigator Consult* |
| High Risk Clinic for Genetic Testing Referral if indicated | High Risk Clinic for Genetic Testing Referral if indicated | High Risk Clinic for Genetic Testing Referral if indicated |
| Surgical Referral per pt/referring physician preference | Surgical Referral per pt/referring physician preference | Surgical Referral per pt/referring physician preference |
| MRI per Surgeon preference +/or Radiology Recommendation | MRI per Surgeon preference +/or Radiology Recommendation | MRI per Surgeon preference +/or Radiology Recommendation |
| Radiation Oncology Referral ALL Lumpectomy Candidates Exception Criteria: ≤ 10mm, low grade, and ≥75 years of age; pt request | Radiation Oncology Referral ALL Lumpectomy Candidates Exception Criteria: ≤ 10mm, low grade, and ≥75 years of age; pt request | Medical Oncology Referral for Post-op Consultation (consider pre-op MedOnc consult for patients needing assistance with surgical decision making) |
| Medical Oncology Referral (Exception Criteria: ≤ 10 mm, low grade, and ≥ 75 years of age) (in cases where neoadjuvant therapy is indicated: locally advanced; lesions ≥ 2 cm; triple negative; Her-2 positive may be scheduled prior to surgeon consult) | Medical Oncology Referral Mastectomy Candidates: Pre-op Lumpectomy Candidates: Surgical Office sets consult for two weeks post- op at time surgery scheduled Exception Criteria: Pt request | |
| Plastic Surgery Referral offered and documented by Surgeon to ALL mastectomy candidates | Plastic Surgery Referral offered and documented by Surgeon to ALL mastectomy candidates | |
| If no pre-op Medical Oncology Referral, Surgical Office sets Medical Oncology consult for two weeks post-op at time surgery is scheduled | | |

*All recommendations based upon National Accreditation Program for Breast Centers (NAPBC) Standards for Accreditation; www.napbc-breast.org

ADH—atypical ductal hyperplasia; ALH—atypical lobular hyperplasia; DCIS—ductal carcinoma in situ; KMC—Kernersville Medical Center; LCIS—lobular carcinoma in situ; MRI—magnetic resonance imaging; NH—Novant Health; pt—patient

*Note.* Figure courtesy of Novant Health Forsyth Medical Center Derrick L. Davis Cancer Center. Used with permission.

## Figure 5-2. Novant Health Greater Winston Breast Nurse Navigator (NHGWBNN) Program Work Flow

**Novant Health Greater Winston Breast Nurse Navigator (NHGWBNN) Program**

⬇

**NHGWBNN Community Outreach**

| NC Northwest Komen Education Committee | Pink Ribbon Talk Committee | Pink Broomstick speaker | Mobile Mamm/CBE | Speak at schools, civic organizations, churches, groups, etc. |

⬇

**All Novant Health Greater Winston Breast Clinic Pathology**

**Benign pathology** – Nurse navigator calls with results and discusses recommendations of the radiologist – 6 month or 1 yr. follow up

**Benign high risk pathology** (atypical ductal hyperplasia, radial scars, papillomas) – Nurse navigator sees patient and arranges surgical follow-up

⬇

**Genetic Clinic offered to all high risk patients**

⬇

**Positive breast cancer pathology**

⬇

**Radiologist shares diagnosis with NHGWBNN present**

All patients referred from outside sources (surgeon, RT, med onc) will be offered NHGWBNN services

⬇

**Patient receives appointment with 1) surgeon, 2) radiation oncologist and/or 3) medical oncologist**

| Breast cancer education | Genetics | Pre-habilitation | Resource specialist | Psychologist | Transportation | Family needs | Neoadjuvant trials |

⬇

NHGWBNN calls patient one week after diagnosis if patient has not been contacted at clinic visit; NHGWBNN calls patient the day after the surgical visit - post-surgery garments are discussed with all mastectomy patients

⬇

**Surgery** (Patient could receive neoadjuvant therapy at this point and loop back into surgery)

⬇

**Call 1 week after surgery**

Are follow up care appointments completed? Continue to assess needs

⬇

Weekly Breast Cancer Multidisciplinary Board to review new cases – clinical trial eligibility discussed on all patients

Navigator selects cases based on pathology or other team members request cases for presentation Information is shared with patient's team after meeting

⬇

Call 3 weeks after surgery Continue to assess needs

Lymphedema Class or 1:1 PT evaluation if needed; prosthesis information reinforced if mastectomy; further surgery for reconstructive needs; clinical trials; Muscles In Motion

⬇

Diet Consult - All triple negatives offered diet consult

⬇

Follow-up Care - Call or meet depending on treatment track

*(Continued on next page)*

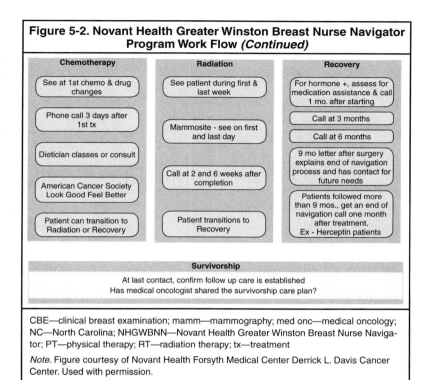

**Figure 5-2. Novant Health Greater Winston Breast Nurse Navigator Program Work Flow** *(Continued)*

| Chemotherapy | Radiation | Recovery |
|---|---|---|
| See at 1st chemo & drug changes | See patient during first & last week | For hormone +, assess for medication assistance & call 1 mo. after starting |
| Phone call 3 days after 1st tx | Mammosite - see on first and last day | Call at 3 months |
| | | Call at 6 months |
| Dietician classes or consult | | 9 mo letter after surgery explains end of navigation process and has contact for future needs |
| American Cancer Society Look Good Feel Better | Call at 2 and 6 weeks after completion | Patients followed more than 9 mos., get an end of navigation call one month after treatment. |
| Patient can transition to Radiation or Recovery | Patient transitions to Recovery | Ex - Herceptin patients |

**Survivorship**

At last contact, confirm follow up care is established
Has medical oncologist shared the survivorship care plan?

CBE—clinical breast examination; mamm—mammography; med onc—medical oncology; NC—North Carolina; NHGWBNN—Novant Health Greater Winston Breast Nurse Navigator; PT—physical therapy; RT—radiation therapy; tx—treatment

*Note.* Figure courtesy of Novant Health Forsyth Medical Center Derrick L. Davis Cancer Center. Used with permission.

Knowing that transportation is a frequent barrier to care, the ONN explores this issue with the patient and discovers that O.W. does drive and has no fear of driving "into the city" for treatment (Clark, Parker, Battaglia, & Freund, 2014). O.W. says she has neighbors and church members who also could help or accompany her, which abate the ONN's social concerns. O.W. feels comfortable leaving her husband when she comes to appointments.

Because of travel distance, the ONN is able to arrange a surgical and radiation oncology visit for O.W. on the same day. Financial resources are discussed. The ONN investigates the possibility of gas cards for the patient through a local cancer support agency and assistance through a cancer center resource specialist (if needed in the future).

Nurse navigators can identify patients who need help with depressive symptoms (Ludman et al., 2015). The ONN notes that

O.W. adamantly stated "no antidepressants." When questioned further, O.W. shares that she does not see the need for antidepressants as long as she can continue her walks and weekly interactions with coworkers and friends. The ONN informs O.W. that counseling is available if needed. Because O.W. takes oral medications for other conditions, compliance is not an immediate concern; however, older adult patients with breast cancer frequently are noncompliant with their hormone therapy (Hershman et al., 2011). The ONN mentions the possibility of hormone therapy. O.W. seems willing to discuss this as a treatment option. The ONN then explains the medical oncologist's role. O.W. has the option of seeing one after surgery; however, team members may decide O.W. needs to see this specialist preoperatively.

Nurse navigators ensure treatment is accomplished based on the National Comprehensive Cancer Network® (NCCN®) guidelines. Genetics play an important role in identifying high-risk individuals (NCCN, 2016). With confirmation by the geneticist, the ONN assesses the Medicare patient as not eligible for testing. O.W. is encouraged to update the healthcare team if additional family history is uncovered.

## What should the role of the ONN be in providing patient education?

Concluding the visit on a positive note, the ONN encourages O.W. to continue walking, working, and participating in other social activities during her preoperative phase of care. The ONN reiterates her availability as well as the availability of financial and counseling support. The ONN also confirms no physical concerns, such as right shoulder immobility or an ambulatory ailment requiring a prehabilitation consult. Prehabilitation consults can be completed by nurse navigators to ensure a patient maintains or improves quality of function (Silver, 2014).

The initial meeting with the ONN supports the findings of Phillips et al. (2014), which demonstrated that a navigator's psychosocial support provided motivation throughout a patient's clinical care, decreased stress with care coordination, and accommodated unbiased listening. The next points of contact with O.W. are a telephone call after her surgery and an in-person visit at the radiation consult (see Figure 5-2).

MammoSite® has been suggested as a radiation treatment option for O.W., as it is an attractive alternative for patients who live far away from radiation facilities. O.W. meets the American Society for Radiation Oncology Consensus Guidelines criteria for this technique (Smith et al., 2009).

The ONN reinforces the teaching on this modality and further questions transportation and overnight housing needs. The ONN suggests the Hospital Hospitality House, a housing facility that is similar to the Ronald McDonald House for pediatric patients. It offers lodging and support to adult patients and their families, providing a compassionate, comfortable alternative to a hospital waiting room or an expensive hotel room for those facing the challenge of out-of-town medical care.

After some thought and discussion with her husband, O.W. chooses the housing option instead of driving daily for the five-day duration of treatment. "I believe my husband and I could use a little vacation," she says.

The ONN meets O.W. and her husband the morning of her surgery to answer last-minute questions and provide support during the sentinel lymph node injection (see Figure 5-2). The ONN visits with O.W. on day 1 of her MammoSite treatments to confirm all housing is in place and to provide needed education and support. The ONN will meet with O.W. again on the last day of treatment to reinforce site care and confirm her understanding of medical oncology follow-up.

O.W. is delighted in her Hospital Hospitality House stay, as she meets many other "interesting people" and "loves the communal evening meals with the other guests."

## What should the ONN do to assist O.W. with her personal survivorship plan of care?

Follow-up calls from the ONN confirm that O.W. has had no skin reactions from her radiation, has seen her medical oncologist in her community setting, and has initiated hormone therapy (see Figure 5-2). She also has not had hot flashes, which can be experienced by more than 70% of breast cancer survivors (Kaplan et al., 2016). O.W. has used exercise (walking) and psychoeducational interventions (job, church) to help her decrease fatigue throughout her care continuum (Mitchell et al., 2016).

Consistent interaction with the ONN after returning to her community shows that O.W. does not have compliance issues with her hormone therapy. Ko et al. (2014) concluded that navigated patients are more likely to receive hormone therapy than non-navigated patients. If noncompliance develops, the ongoing relationship between the ONN and O.W. provides an opportunity to explore the root causes and offer resources to help overcome the barriers (Shockney, 2013).

## Summary and Key Points

Breast cancer occurrence in older adults is increasing; ensuring this population receives the best quality care should be a shared priority of the healthcare team (Muss, 2011). O.W. was an older adult patient with breast cancer who started her breast cancer screening in her local community, went to a larger cancer center for her acute breast cancer care, and circled back to her community for long-term follow-up. Navigation was the bridge that connected the individual patient to her community and available medical resources and support. Fillion and colleagues (2012) described the work of nurse navigation as bidimensional—patient centered and health system oriented. O.W. was evaluated on a personal level with respect to her physical age versus her chronologic age. Consistent contact by the ONN, either in person or by telephone, allowed O.W. to evolve through the necessary healthcare team interactions and to use available resources to support transitions through her personalized care journey. O.W. was highly satisfied with her care, even suggesting ways her church group could help the Hospital Hospitality House with house items or meals.

- Breast cancer occurrence in older adults is increasing. Half of women who are diagnosed with breast cancer will be aged 61 or older (American Cancer Society, 2015).
- Breast nurse navigators can perform patient-centered education on breast cancer type and possible treatment options. They also can be available during the disease trajectory to proactively guide patients through care transitions with additional education and support (Pedersen & Hack, 2010).
- The navigator's psychosocial support throughout the patient's clinical care provides motivation and decreases stress with care

coordination by incorporating unbiased listening (Phillips et al., 2014).

- Navigated patients are more likely to receive hormone therapy than non-navigated patients (Ko et al., 2014).

## Questions

### What is one action that an older adult woman can take to decrease the risk of dying from breast cancer?

An action an older adult woman can take to decrease the risk of dying from breast cancer is to participate in routine mammography screenings (Lauby-Secretan et al., 2015).

### What can greatly influence a patient with breast cancer who is receiving hormone therapy?

Patient navigation can have a direct influence on a patient with breast cancer receiving hormone therapy.

## References

American Cancer Society. (2015). *Breast cancer facts and figures 2015–2016*. Retrieved from http://http://www.cancer.org/acs/groups/content/@research/documents/document/acspc-046381.pdf

Boa, T., & Davidson, N.E. (2008). Gene expression profiling of breast cancer. *Advances in Surgery, 42*, 249–260. doi:10.1016/j.yasu.2008.03.002

Clark, J.A., Parker, V.A., Battaglia, T.A., & Freund, K.M. (2014). Patterns of task and network actions performed by navigators to facilitate cancer care. *Health Care Management Review, 39*, 90–101. doi:10.1097/HMR.0b013e31828da41e

Desimini, E.M., Kennedy, J.A., Helsley, M.F., Denton, C., Rice, T.T., Stannard, B., ... Lewis, M.G. (2011). Making the case for nurse navigators—Benefits, outcomes, and return on investment. *Oncology Issues, 26*(5), 26–33. Retrieved from http://pages.nxtbook.com/nxtbooks/accc/oncologyissues_20110910/offline/accc_oncologyissues_20110910.pdf

Fillion, L., Cook, S., Veillette, A.-N., Aubin, M., de Serres, M., Rainville, F., ... Doll, R. (2012). Professional navigation framework: Elaboration and validation in a Canadian context [Online exclusive]. *Oncology Nursing Forum, 39*, E58–E69. doi:10.1188/12.ONF.E58-E69

Hershman, D.L., Shao, T., Kushi, L.H., Buono, D., Tsai, W.Y., Fehrenbacher, L., ... Neugut, A.I. (2011). Early discontinuation and non-adherence to adjuvant hormonal therapy are associated with increased mortality in women with breast cancer. *Breast Cancer Research and Treatment, 126*, 529–537. doi:10.1007/s10549-010-1132-4

Kaplan, M., Carpenter, J., Abernathy, E., Fernandez-Ortega, M.P., Foster, J., Grimmer, D., & Mahon, S. (2016). Putting evidence into practice: Hot flashes. Retrieved from https://www.ons.org/practice-resources/pep/hot-flashes

Ko, N.Y., Darnell, J.S., Calhoun, E., Freund, K.M., Wells, K.J., Shapiro, C.L., ... Battaglia, T.A. (2014). Can patient navigation improve receipt of recommended breast cancer care? Evidence from the National Patient Research Program. *Journal of Clinical Oncology, 32*, 2758–2764. doi:10.1200/JCO.2013.53.6037

Lauby-Secretan, B., Scoccianti, C., Loomis, D., Benbrahim-Tallaa, L., Bouvard, V., Bianchini, F., ... Straif, K. (2015). Breast-cancer screening—Viewpoint of the IARC Working Group. *New England Journal of Medicine, 372*, 2353–2358. doi:10.1056/NEJMsr1504363

Ludman, E.J., McCorkle, R., Bowles, E.A., Rutter, C.M., Chubak, J., Tuzzio, L., ... Wagner, E.H. (2015). Do depressed newly diagnosed cancer patients differentially benefit from nurse navigation? *General Hospital Psychiatry, 37*, 236–239. doi:10.1016/j.genhosppsych.2015.02.008

Mitchell, S.A., Alkaiyat, M.O., Clark, J.C., DeGennaro, R.M., Hoffman, A.J., Huenerberg, K., ... Weisbrod, B.M. (2016). Putting evidence into practice: Fatigue. Retrieved from https://www.ons.org/practice-resources/pep/fatigue

Muss, H.B. (2011). Older women with breast cancer: Slow progress, great opportunity, now is the time. *Journal of Clinical Oncology, 29*, 4608–4610. doi:10.1200/JCO.2011.38.6888

National Comprehensive Cancer Network. (2016). *NCCN Clinical Practice Guidelines in Oncology (NCCN Guidelines®): Genetic/familial high-risk assessment: Breast and ovarian* [v.2.2016]. Retrieved from http://www.nccn.org/professionals/physician_gls/pdf/genetics_screening.pdf

Pederson, A., & Hack, T.F. (2010). Pilots of oncology health care: A concept analysis of the patient navigator role. *Oncology Nursing Forum, 37*, 55–60. doi:10.1188/10.ONF.55-60

Phillips, S., Nonzee, N., Tom, L., Murphy, K., Hajjar, N., Bularzik, C., ... Simon, M.A. (2014). Patient navigators' reflections on the navigator-patient relationship. *Journal of Cancer Education, 29*, 337–344. doi:10.1007/s13187-014-0612-3

Shockney, L. (2013). Medication nonadherence: Causes and solutions [Webinar]. Retrieved from https://www.aonnonline.org/education/interactive-learning

Silver, J.K. (2014). Cancer prehabilitation and its role in improving health outcomes and reducing health care costs. *Seminars in Oncology Nursing, 31*, 13–30. doi:10.1016/j.soncn.2014.11.003

Smith, B.D., Arthur, D.W., Buchholz, T.A., Haffty, B.G., Hahn, C.A., Hardenbergh, P.H., ... Harris, J.R. (2009). Accelerated partial breast irradiation consensus statement from the American Society for Radiation Oncology (ASTRO). *International Journal of Radiation Oncology, Biology, Physics, 74*, 987–1001. doi:10.1016/j.ijrobp.2009.02.031

# CASE 6
# Metastatic Breast Cancer

Lillie D. Shockney, RN, BS, MAS

J.B. is a 32-year-old woman who reports right hip and lower back pain. She was originally diagnosed with stage IIB invasive ductal cancer in her left breast almost three years ago. She has been married for seven years and has two young boys, aged 3 and 4. J.B. is a stay-at-home mom and does volunteer work for her church. She declined genetic counseling and testing when originally diagnosed, as no history of breast cancer existed in her family. At that time, her American Joint Committee on Cancer (AJCC) staging information from surgical pathology was T2 N1 M0. The tumor was a 4 cm (T2) sentinel lymph node biopsy (N1) when tested pretreatment. Based on scans performed as part of the staging workup, no evidence was found that the cancer had spread to distant sites (M0).

## What is the role of the oncology nurse navigator (ONN) in a newly diagnosed patient with breast cancer?

In J.B.'s first meeting with her ONN after her original diagnosis, she was asked about her life goals. J.B. did not plan on having more children; therefore, fertility preservation was not factored into the treatment planning process. Her goals included raising her two young boys, becoming a leader in her church, and possibly returning to college after her sons enter middle school. The ONN discovered that J.B.'s career interest is in theology and that her husband works full-time at a local grocery store in a management position. In conducting a needs assessment, the ONN found no barriers to J.B. getting treatments as prescribed (see Figure 6-1).

## Figure 6-1. Potential Problems/Barriers to Care

This list is to be used to help you to identify patient concerns at the initial visit and at each follow-up visit. It will help you develop a plan of action, including referrals to appropriate departments.

**Health Insurance/Financial Concerns**
• Inadequate or lack of insurance coverage
• Precertification problems
• Difficulty paying bills
• Need for financial assistance from Medicaid/Medicare
• Confusing financial paperwork
• Need for prescription assistance
• Need for medical equipment or supplies (wheelchairs, dressings)
• Citizenship problems/undocumented status
• Other: _____

**Transportation To and From Treatment**
• Public transportation needed
• Private transportation needed
• Ambulette (independent ambulance transportation) services required
• Other: _____

**Physical Needs**
• Child/elder care
• Housing/housing problems
• Food, clothing, other physical needs
• Prostheses, wigs, etc.
• Vocational support (job skills, employment skills)
• Extended care needs: home care, hospice, long-term care
• Other: _____

**Communication/Cultural Needs**
• Primary language other than English
• Inability to read/write
• Poor health literacy
• Cultural barriers (i.e., effect on lifestyle choices)
• Other: _____

**Disease Management**
• Treatment compliance issues (missed appointments, unwillingness to take medicine)
• Needs help with obtaining a second opinion (if desired by patient)
• Mental health services needed
• Does not understand treatment plan and/or procedures
• Needs to talk to provider (physician, nurse, therapist, etc.)

*(Continued on next page)*

| **Figure 6-1. Potential Problems/Barriers to Care *(Continued)*** |
|---|
| • Wants more information about:_____<br>• Other:_____<br>*[Note to Navigator: Add to this list as you encounter other barriers to care. Below is a list of support services. You may need to suggest that the patient ask his or her health care provider about a referral.]*<br><br>**Supportive Services for Referrals**<br>• Social workers<br>• Clergy<br>• Nutritionists<br>• Genetic counselors<br>• Financial counselors<br>• Physical, occupational, and speech therapists<br>• Psychologists<br>• Board-certified psychiatrists specializing in hospice/palliative medicine |
| *Note.* From *Cancer Patient Navigation Program Toolkit* (pp. 19–20), by Kansas Cancer Partnership, 2009. Retrieved from http://www.cancerkansas.org/download/Cancer _Patient_Navigation_Toolkit.pdf. Reprinted with permission. |

J.B.'s original treatments included neoadjuvant chemotherapy of doxorubicin, cyclophosphamide, and paclitaxel. She was very ill during these treatments, requiring hospitalization for neutropenia once and IV hydration as an outpatient twice.

The primary breast tumor did not shrink. Her tumor was moderately estrogen receptor positive (60%), progesterone receptor negative (0%), and HER2 negative. Following a left-modified radical mastectomy surgery with tissue expander insertion performed three weeks after completion of a doxorubicin, cyclophosphamide, and paclitaxel (ACT) chemotherapy regimen, J.B. underwent radiation to the left chest wall and axilla. Three positive nodes out of a total of 12 were surgically removed. Given that J.B. was premenopausal, she was placed on tamoxifen as hormonal therapy after radiation therapy was completed.

Eight months after treatment, J.B. planned on permanent reconstruction in the form of a deep inferior epigastric perforator flap; however, she chose to delay this due to summer vacation and other pressing church-based responsibilities.

She was taking tamoxifen as prescribed daily but was experiencing problems with hot flashes and night sweats. These symptoms were causing J.B. difficulty with getting a good night's sleep, which affected her ability to function effectively as a mother.

Just nine months following completion of her radiation, J.B. begins to have right hip pain and lower back pain. She is seen by her medical oncologist, who does a new staging workup, including a positron-emission tomography–computed tomography scan, bone scan, and CA27-29 tumor marker. Findings show lesions in her upper-right femur near the head of the acetabulum and lumbar vertebras 3, 4, and 5 of her spine. Suspicious areas are found in her lungs. One lesion (2 cm) looks questionable in her liver. Her tumor marker is 68. She is informed by her medical oncologist that the cause of her lower back and hip pain is the development of metastatic breast cancer.

## How can the ONN educate this patient?

J.B. asks her ONN, "How can breast cancer have grown that quickly in my bones, liver, and lungs? My scans looked fine before."

The ONN explains that scans are not able to show microscopic diseases that may be present within other organs. In such a case, the cancer likely was already present but too small to see on the original staging. When breast cancer does spread to other organs and is invasive ductal carcinoma, it commonly travels to the bones, liver, or lungs. The ONN reaffirms to J.B. that she did all of the treatments recommended to her for the purpose of preventing metastatic disease. However, these treatments do not always work.

J.B. asks, "Can you refer me to a surgeon who can just cut the cancers out of these organs—the same as what was done with my breast and lymph nodes?"

Sometimes, an isolated small liver metastasis can be ablated or surgically removed (Meloni et al., 2009). The ONN explains that, due to the diffuse nature of the cancer, this likely is not feasible.

The ONN explains that the first step is to perform a biopsy of one or several of these lesions to confirm metastatic breast cancer and to evaluate the prognostic factors of the metastatic disease. This must happen before a treatment plan can be determined (Sighoko, Liu, Hou, Gustafson, & Huo, 2014; Yang, Liao, Peng, Xie, & Xie, 2014).

J.B. asks, "Would the hormone receptor and HER2 not be the same, as they were in the tumor in my breast and lymph nodes?"

The ONN explains that, for metastatic breast cancer, it is scientifically proven that these receptors can sometimes change and become the opposite of what they originally were when the primary tumor was tested in pathology (Ieni et al., 2014; Qu et al., 2014).

A biopsy of the lung and the bone are performed, confirming the presence of breast cancer cells. These cells are now 0% estrogen receptor positive. HER2 remains negative. The multidisciplinary team decides that J.B.'s treatment will be a randomized, open-label, multicenter phase III clinical trial—cisplatin plus gemcitabine versus paclitaxel plus gemcitabine as first-line therapy for metastatic triple-negative breast cancer (CBCSG006).

J.B. is randomized to receive cisplatin plus gemcitabine (Hu et al., 2015). She feels she should be given "stronger medications." The ONN explains that the purpose of treatment now is to control the disease and treat it like a chronic illness. The mission is not curative this time. The treatments need to preserve quality of life while controlling the cancer to whatever degree possible. This is still hard to accept for J.B., as she feels she has done all she can to prevent metastatic disease. The ONN arranges for J.B. to talk with another young mother receiving similar treatments for metastatic disease. J.B. also is directed to the Metastatic Breast Cancer Network's website (www.mbcn.org) for support and resources.

## How can the ONN help the patient and her husband identify goals moving forward?

The ONN says, "Let's revisit your life goals from before. When you were first diagnosed a few years ago, your goals were to raise your boys and get more involved with your church, including becoming a church leader. I recall you telling me about a desire to return to school to study theology. Are these still your life goals?"

J.B. confirms her goals, but now she worries that she will not see her children grow into adulthood. She wants hard and fast survival statistics and assurance that she will be alive for decades to come. The ONN explains that there are no guarantees and that it is best to first see how the cancer responds to these new treatments. Some patients live a short time, while others live for several decades. J.B. says that her husband has told her that she "cannot die" because he cannot raise their children on his own. The ONN speaks with the husband, making him aware that saying such things places added burden on his wife. She has no personal control over this disease and how it will or will not be able to be controlled in the future.

The ONN also tells the couple that there likely will be additional goals that J.B. will want to adopt or consider in the future. The ONN also encourages J.B. to tap into her spiritual resources for support by making her church friends aware of her new diagnosis. Although the goal of treatment is not curative, giving and receiving hope remains important (Bouleuc & Chvetzoff, 2009; Shockney, 2014). A primary focus should be on the patient's goals.

"It is appropriate to be optimistic for as long as it is realistic, but you should always have a backup plan when the time comes to make end-of-life plans," the ONN tells J.B. and her husband.

J.B. gets underway with her treatments, which consist of radiation to her hip and spine. Her bone pain is greatly alleviated. She also receives cisplatin plus gemcitabine as part of a clinical trial. She has scans done three months into her new treatments for metastatic breast cancer. The metastatic lesion in her liver is much smaller and her metastatic bone disease also has minimized.

Once again, no barriers to care exist until well into J.B.'s treatment, when her husband's insurance at work changes. Unlike his previous insurance, this insurance has high deductibles and co-payments. The ONN is able to get the patient financial support through drug discount programs available from pharmaceutical companies and through organizations such as the Red Devils (www.the-red-devils.org) and the Patient Advocate Foundation (www.patientadvocate.org). These organizations help cover J.B.'s household bills, allowing her to pay the bills not covered her by insurance.

## How can the ONN discuss opportunities for metastatic breast cancer activities?

Three months into J.B.'s treatment, the ONN tells J.B. and her husband about a metastatic breast cancer retreat. They express interest and register to attend the next retreat, occurring in two months.

About five months into her treatment, J.B.'s cancer status changes. She begins experiencing pronounced fatigue with evidence of ascites developing. Her scans show that the cancer in her liver is growing. She also develops dyspnea on exertion and pleural effusion, which requires a thoracentesis. About 1,200 ml of fluid is siphoned from her pleural cavities. Current treatments are stopped. The oncologist plans a meeting with J.B. in one week to discuss further drug options.

At this point, the ONN asks J.B., "What is your greatest concern?"

With these pronounced changes and her cancer becoming more aggressive, J.B. is worried about how much time she has left with her children. She states, "I now have two specific goals. One is to have as much quality time with my children as I can. I want to live long enough for them to remember me. The other is to receive chemotherapy up until my last breath. I want my husband and mother to be able to tell my boys that I fought to be with them."

The ONN reminds the couple of the upcoming metastatic breast cancer survivor retreat. They are preregistered and have arranged child care for their boys. The retreat is three days and two nights. It provides couples dealing with a metastatic breast cancer diagnosis the ability to network and discuss their concerns in small group sessions and in private. Couples can develop coping skills and a better understanding of what to expect regarding treatment, allowing them to proactively prepare for what lies ahead and to learn about research efforts that provide hope for future generations. They also can develop better ways of managing stress and communicating with each other, their oncology specialists, and their children.

Both J.B. and her husband feel it would helpful for them to attend. The ONN explains that she will be running this retreat with two other ONNs. There will even be some fun during the event, including playing the "Almost Newly Wed Game." The ONN advises that the retreat requires their undivided attention and that cell phones will be turned off (except at bedtime to tell their boys good night). This is the couple's time to be together and to spend time with others in similar circumstances. The ONN will confirm with J.B.'s medical oncologist if she is stable enough to attend and participate.

At the retreat, the ONN presents all 12 couples with a profound question: "Of everything that lies ahead, what is your greatest fear?"

The couples are divided into different rooms. Patients are placed in one room. Their spouses or partners are placed in another. A primary concern among those with young children is a feeling that they will not be around to raise them. They fear they will miss specific and significant milestones in their lives.

J.B. speaks about her two goals—wanting to spend quality time with her boys and wanting to receive chemotherapy up to her last breath. The ONN tells J.B. that these two goals actually conflict with one another. The ONN explains that if J.B. opts for treatment until her last breath, she should expect to be quite ill, likely warranting hospitalization. Her boys would be too young to be in the hospital. They could be psychologically harmed by seeing their ill mother with tubes and IVs in a hospital bed. By opting for hospice care sooner versus later, J.B. likely would live longer. She would be able to spend more time with her children and have a better remaining quality of life (Morrogh et al., 2010; Rugno, Paiva, & Paiva, 2014).

## What is the ONN's role in navigating primary care from the medical oncologist to the palliative care team?

At the encouragement of the ONN, J.B. and her husband request a consultation with the palliative care team as well as a discussion in their home with a hospice coordinator. With the ONN's help, they prepare for the discussion with the oncologist by looking at all options, including stopping treatment in favor of symptom management and receiving palliative care and hospice care at home. By doing so, J.B. and her husband better understand how best to prepare for what likely lies ahead, how symptom management will be addressed to preserve quality of life, and how to make decisions considering hospice care. Instead of feeling a sense of fear or uncertainty, they now are developing a sense of control— not over the cancer, but over how J.B. wishes to live the remainder of her life. Literature is provided on how to talk with young children about this process.

At the retreat, J.B. is given the opportunity to select greeting cards for each of her sons. These cards associate with milestones her children likely will reach without her physical presence. She picks cards for celebrating birthdays, receiving communion, getting driver's licenses, graduating from high school and college, getting married, and even having children. The idea is that J.B. will write what she would say to her children if she were to be physically able to be present during these events. By writing these cards, she can still be "there" during these events, instilling her hope, love, and wisdom into her children. J.B. also is given recordable children's books, allowing her to record her voice reading to her young boys.

J.B. now is relying a lot on her faith to sustain her. She hopes to die with dignity at home with her family. She discusses her concern that her husband is not at the same point of acceptance. The ONN arranges for a pro bono psychotherapist to support him.

After the retreat, a plan is created for J.B.'s husband that will provide him and the children support during J.B.'s hospice care and after her death. In addition, the ONN connects J.B.'s mother with Mothers Supporting Daughters with Breast Cancer (www.mothers daughters.org). This organization provides one-on-one support to mothers via mother volunteers, including those who have lost daughters to breast cancer. J.B. and her husband are encouraged to continue to reach out to their church for support. The ONN also provides them with contact information for a pro bono videographer. Similar to the greeting cards, a video can provide J.B. an outlet to speak to her boys after her passing. She can film herself telling her boys that she loves them or even what she wishes for their futures.

## How can the ONN assist J.B. and her family?

The ONN also discusses the elements of experiencing a "good death" with J.B. and her husband. Having a "good death" includes knowing you had purpose for living and that you were valued by at least one other person, leaving a legacy that does not mean just leaving money, giving forgiveness and receiving forgiveness, knowing you will be spoken of fondly after you are gone, being pain free, leaving no bad debt associated with your cancer treatment, feeling a spiritual connection to a higher power, and fulfilling some specific life goals while here and alternatively after you are gone (Shockney, 2014).

During J.B.'s illness, she has taken several online theology courses. She also has become a Sunday school teacher. Some of the lesson plans she has developed have been to help young children understand that a parent's illness is not the child's fault. She also has spent time journaling about the things she has learned from her children through this journey, including how little things become big things to celebrate, how each hour with them has been a gift, and how she has found answers through prayer. She also has written that treatment for treatment's sake is not good treatment, documenting her dilemma of making goals that conflict with one another. She has written future notes to her husband, to her boys, and to her potential grandchildren.

The ONN identifies additional resources for the patient and her family, which include an art therapy program for young children to express their emotions and worries. The ONN serves as the patient advocate, ensuring the patient's goals are the focus of her care and preventing J.B. from getting treatment for treatment's sake. The navigator also encourages J.B.'s mother to reach out to church membership to request assistance with babysitting, meal delivery, and running errands for the family, allowing for their finances to remain in control as best as possible and the family to spend as much time together as they can.

After extensive discussions with the medical oncologist and palliative care oncologist, J.B. has chosen not to receive chemotherapy and to enroll in hospice care. While difficult for J.B.'s treatment team, mother, and husband, the ONN reiterates the importance of respecting J.B.'s wishes after confirming the patient understands her options.

J.B. receives hospice care at home for four months. With the ONN's assistance, her husband applies for the Family and Medical Leave Act, allowing him more time with his wife. After receiving coaching from the ONN on how to talk with his supervisor about his family's needs, the husband is able to get a more flexible schedule during this period of time. The ONN also provides him with books to help explain to his children what is happening to their mother. Although he struggles with his anger that his wife is "being stolen away from him," he is able to recognize that it is not helpful to vent these thoughts to her. Through continued counseling, he is able to reach a point of acceptance, though never to the level that J.B. personally reaches through her spirituality.

J.B. truly gets closure with her family, other loved ones, and herself. She is content that her husband will do a good job with the boys, especially with assistance from his sister and her mother. Her spiritual awareness gives her confidence that she will serve as a guardian angel for her family. She even is able to write a letter to her husband telling him to fall in love again, believing it a waste of his love if he were to remain unmarried. The ONN provides J.B., her husband, and her mother with a list of elements that make up a "good death"

(Shockney, 2014). Each element is discussed, along with plans on how to accomplish them.

Parts of J.B.'s legacy are her Sunday school lesson plans and her journal of wisdom learned from a mother of young children.

## Summary and Key Points

There is no time more vulnerable in a patient's life than when faced with a diagnosis of metastatic breast cancer. The ONN has a pivotal and profound role in supporting such patients and their families. This begins with patient education about what such a diagnosis means and how treatment for metastatic breast cancer is approached differently compared to earlier and curable cancers. These patients have life goals, just as those patients who will survive and thrive after treatment is completed. The ONN can provide emotional support and guidance that goes beyond traditional navigation functions, including helping patients and their families to fulfill life goals and future hopes in alternative ways, facilitating the patient and their spouse or partner to attend a retreat designed for those with dealing with metastatic disease, helping patients' voices become heard concerning their goals as treatment is planned and given, and doing whatever possible to facilitate the elements of a "good death."

- Patient education is a primary responsibility of the ONN. It must be provided across the continuum of care and frequently reiterated. Education includes translating terminology, explaining the philosophy of goals of treatment for early-stage versus late-stage disease, and discussing treatment phases and how decisions will be made with the patient.
- Patients have life goals that they will not be able to personally fulfill. The ONN needs to assist in creating alternative ways for patients and their families to fulfill these goals and hopes after the patient is gone.
- Identification of barriers to care and resources to undo these barriers is a primary responsibility of the ONN. Barriers in communication can also exist, especially when dealing with patients with end-stage disease who may be confused about what treatments are intended to do for them.
- Metastatic breast cancer couples retreats are available at several locations nationally and are a valuable resource for patients and

their partners to experience, giving them the opportunity to meet others with the same clinical situation, develop new coping skills, discuss fears, learn about clinical trials, hear about the future solutions for the next generation, and begin the process of getting affairs in order and fulfilling the elements of a good death experience.

- Transitioning from the medical oncologist to the palliative care team and hospice services can be difficult, as patients can feel abandoned by the medical oncology team providing treatment. The ONN is critically important during this transition in educating patients and their families about the goals of care and that palliative care focuses on symptom management and preservation or restoration of quality of life.
- The ONN remaining in touch with the patient and family once hospice is initiated is helpful in keeping a bridge between the prior treatment team and the new care team.
- Nothing can be more fulfilling to ONNs than knowing that they helped a patient experience a "good death" and that they prepared the family to continue their lives without the patient while helping to preserve their memory and simultaneously fulfilling the patient's future goals and hopes.

## Questions

### What is a nonprofit organization that provides financial support to patients with metastatic breast cancer?

A nonprofit organization that provides financial support for patients with metastatic breast cancer is the Patient Advocate Foundation (www.patientadvocate.org).

### What are the elements of a "good death?"

The elements of a "good death" are knowing you had purpose for living and that you are valued by at least one other person, leaving a legacy that does not mean just leaving money, giving forgiveness and receiving forgiveness, knowing you will be spoken of fondly after you are gone, being pain free, leaving no bad debt associated with your cancer treatment, feeling a spiritual connection to a higher power, and fulfilling some specific life goals while here in alternative ways after you are gone (Shockney, 2014).

# References

Bouleuc, C., & Chvetzoff, G. (2009). End of chemotherapy decision for metastatic breast cancer patients. *Bulletin du Cancer, 96*(Suppl. 2), 81–89.

Hu, X.-C., Zhang, J., Xu, B.-H., Cai, L., Ragaz, J., Wang, Z.-H., … Shao, Z.M. (2015). Cisplatin plus gemcitabine versus paclitaxel plus gemcitabine as first-line therapy for metastatic triple-negative breast cancer (CBCSG006): A randomized, open-label, multicentre, phase 3 trial. *Lancet Oncology, 16,* 436–446. doi:10.1016/S1470 -2045(15)70064-1

Ieni, A., Barresi, V., Caltabiano, R., Cascone, A.M., Del Sordo, R., Cabibi, D., … Tuccari, G. (2014). Discordance rate of HER2 status in primary breast carcinoma versus synchronous axillary lymph node metastases: A multicenter retrospective investigation. *OncoTargets and Therapy, 11,* 1267–1272. doi:10.2147/OTT.S65294

Meloni, M.F., Andreano, A., Laeseke, P.F., Livraghi, T., Sironi, S., & Lee, F.T., Jr. (2009). Breast cancer liver metastases: US-guided percutaneous radiofrequency ablation—intermediate and long-term survival rates. *Radiology, 253,* 861–869. doi:10.1148/radiol.2533081968

Morrogh, M., Miner, T.J., Park, A., Jenckes, A., Gonen, M., Seidman, A., … King, T.A. (2010). A prospective evaluation of the durability of palliative interventions for patients with metastatic breast cancer. *Cancer, 116,* 3338–3347. doi:10.1002/ cncr.25034

Qu, Q., Zong, Y., Fei, X.-C., Chen, X.S., Xu, C., Lou, G.-Y., & Shen, K.-W. (2014). The importance of biopsy in clinically diagnosed metastatic lesions in patients with breast cancer. *World Journal of Surgical Oncology, 12,* 93. doi:10.1186/1477-7819 -12-93

Rugno, F.C., Paiva, B.S., & Paiva, C.E. (2014). Early integration of palliative care facilitates the discontinuation of anticancer treatment in women with advanced breast or gynecologic cancers. *Gynecologic Oncology, 135,* 249–254. doi:10.1016/j. ygyno.2014.08.030

Shockney, L.D. (2014). *Fulfilling hope: Supporting the needs of patients with advanced cancers.* New York, NY: Nova Science Publishers.

Sighoko, D., Liu, J., Hou, N., Gustafson, P., & Huo, D. (2014). Discordance in hormone receptor status among primary, metastatic, and second primary breast cancers: Biological differences or misclassification? *Oncologist, 19,* 592–601. doi:10.1634/theoncologist.2013-0427

Yang, Y.-F., Liao, Y.-Y., Peng, N.-F., Xie, S.-R., & Xie, Y.-F. (2014). Discordances in ER, PR and HER2 receptors between primary and recurrent/metastatic lesions and their impact on survival in breast cancer patients. *Medical Oncology, 31,* 214. doi:10.1007/s12032-014-0214-2

# CASE 7
# Navigating a Young Patient

Barbara Francks, RN, BSN, OCN®, CBCN®

J.K. is a 25-year-old G1P1 mother who has discovered a small lump in her right breast. She has felt this lump for three months but had thought it was related to her menstrual cycle. Noting a change in the lump, she seeks evaluation by her gynecologist.

A diagnostic mammogram and ultrasound reveals a density in her right breast. J.K. is referred to a breast surgeon. On examination, a 2.5 cm tumor is palpated in her right breast as well as a single firm axillary node in the axillae. An ultrasound-guided core biopsy of the primary site and the lymph node is performed, which reveals a poorly differentiated invasive ductal carcinoma, estrogen receptor 0%, progesterone receptor 0%, and HER2 negative. Her magnetic resonance imaging (MRI) is negative. The results are thoroughly discussed with J.K. and her husband at a follow-up appointment with the surgeon and the oncology nurse navigator (ONN). After discussing the findings, J.K. is referred to the multidisciplinary oncology team. This team approach is very important to achieving successful patient outcomes.

J.K. and her husband meet with the multidisciplinary team, which includes a plastic surgeon, a medical oncologist and radiation oncologist, a clinical trials screening nurse, a genetic counselor, and a fertility specialist. The ONN reassures J.K. and her husband that she will be in close communication, assisting in scheduling appointments and coordinating J.K.'s care. J.K. is given a breast cancer journey notebook, which provides information, resources, and a place to keep important healthcare information.

After a long and emotional meeting, J.K. and her husband appear overwhelmed. The ONN recommends contacting her the next day to schedule appointments and further discuss J.K.'s journey. This allows the couple an opportunity to process the information and formulate questions. The ONN achieves her goals for this initial encounter—to meet the patient and her husband, assess immediate needs, and establish a supportive interaction to begin the foundation for a therapeutic relationship.

The next day, the ONN answers J.K.'s questions. J.K. then has the following concerns:

- "How will I care for and parent my three-year-old son with numerous upcoming appointments and treatments?"
- "What about my future plans of having another child and advancing in my career?"
- "Will I be here to watch my child (and future children) grow to adulthood?"

Additionally, J.K. expresses concern about future treatment decisions. Finances are a great concern to the family, as J.K.'s husband receives an hourly wage and missing work would be a huge burden on their finances. Also, the family has very little support from relatives. J.K. expresses feeling overwhelmed and "not in control."

## What can the ONN do to provide support to J.K. and her husband?

- Actively listen to J.K.'s concerns to better understand how the diagnosis and treatment will affect J.K. and her family.
- Provide reassurance by helping J.K. feel confident that problems are understood and will be addressed.
- Provide a safe environment to air frustrations. J.K. expresses that it is essential for her to maintain a normal life and family routine, minimizing disruption from treatment as much as possible. This is acknowledged and noted by the ONN and will be shared with the medical team as an important goal for J.K.
- Refer to social work to provide counseling and support.
- Provide ongoing education related to J.K.'s disease and plan of care.

## What consults need to be arranged by the ONN for J.K.?

- Reproductive medicine to discuss fertility options
- Genetic counseling
- Medical oncology to discuss chemotherapy option

- Appointments with a plastic surgeon and radiation oncologist. Scheduling appointments early is important for making decisions, optimizing treatment delivery, and minimizing risks (Reyna & Lee, 2014).

The ONN provides ongoing education and a review of the plan of care. J.K.'s journey notebook includes tools for her to use at her consults. These tools are discussed and personalized to better meet J.K.'s needs for gathering information and, ultimately, making decisions.

J.K.'s genetic risk assessment shows no significant family history, but given her young age as well as her triple-negative histology, which is associated with an increased risk to carry a *BRCA* mutation, genetic testing is recommended (National Cancer Institute, 2016). No mutations are found on genetic testing; however, J.K. will need further discussions with her care team before making an informed surgical decision.

The medical oncologist recommends chemotherapy with four cycles of dose-dense doxorubicin and cyclophosphamide with growth factor support. This will be followed by 12 weekly cycles of paclitaxel. There will be no role for antiestrogen therapy.

The medical oncologist also discusses options for adjuvant versus neoadjuvant chemotherapy and clinical trial eligibility. Studies show that triple-negative breast cancer responds well in the neoadjuvant setting, with higher pathologic complete response compared to other breast tumor types (von Minckwitz & Martin, 2012).

J.K. understands that receiving chemotherapy before surgery does not affect survival; however, it can change the timing of treatment as well as surgical options (von Minckwitz & Martin, 2012). It is made clear to J.K. that this treatment, given to destroy cancer cells, will also affect other cells, organs, and hormones and possibly interfere with her fertility.

> **What steps should the ONN take to help J.K. make informed decisions regarding fertility and other long-term life goals?**

After receiving reproductive counseling and hearing their options, J.K. and her husband elect not to pursue fertility preservation. The ONN explains the importance of gathering similar information and careful planning in making informed choices and optimizing future outcomes and overall quality of life. Although J.K. says she understands, she is beginning to realize the influence of cancer and its treatment on every aspect of her life. It is the ONN's goal to engage the patient and her husband as integral members of the care team, actively involving them by educating and imparting information to help them come to decisions and achieve their goals. J.K.'s informed preferences are sought and respected by the care team.

## What role does the ONN play once J.K.'s treatment begins?

J.K. meets with the breast surgeon to finalize a treatment plan. She will receive neoadjuvant chemotherapy. The role of radiation will be determined based on surgical decision and postoperative pathologic findings. J.K. expresses both confidence and relief in her decision and is ready to move forward with treatment.

Once treatment is initiated and underway, the ONN visits the patient at the infusion center and, on occasion, provides items donated by local organizations, such as hats, scarves, and small gift bags. These seemingly small items make a big difference to J.K., as they show the compassion and never-wavering support of the ONN, who is continually assessing resources and supportive needs.

## How does the ONN assist J.K. concerning financial resources?

J.K. is interested in learning more about financial resources listed in her journey notebook. She completes several grant applications, which the ONN submits for her. Financial support for child care is received. Other local organizations assist in the payment of several late utility bills. During the holidays, the ONN refers the family to an organization that provides holiday gifts, which are gratefully received by each family member.

## How does the ONN support J.K. during the surgery process?

J.K. has a good clinical response to her chemotherapy treatments. Options for surgery are presented. In general, patients underestimate how surgical decisions will influence postoperative quality of life. Reyna and Lee (2014) reported that women under the age of 50 have an average of 0.1% risk for contralateral breast cancer (CBC); however, a diagnosis under the age of 45 doubles that risk. A contralateral prophylactic mastectomy may reduce the risk of CBC, but no evidence exists of survival benefit (Davies, Cantor, & Brewster, 2015).

In a follow-up phone call with her ONN, J.K. shares the outcome of her visit. J.K. identifies symmetry and fear of recurrence as reasons for her decision to opt for bilateral mastectomy with reconstruction. Although she has been informed of the alternatives and that symmetry can be achieved through other means by her plastic surgeon, J.K. expresses confidence with her choice. Radiation is still an unknown factor, and autologous reconstruction is recommended using a deep inferior epigastric perforator flap, for which J.K. is a good candidate. Use of J.K.'s own tissue will improve cosmetic outcomes if radiation is needed.

The ONN meets with the couple preoperatively, providing verbal, visual, and written education materials and using a return demonstration (teach-back method) during all education opportunities.

Preparing for surgery is an emotional time. J.K. expresses fear and concern about how this surgery will affect her self-image, sexuality, and the quality of her marital relationship. She is receptive to speaking with an oncology social worker to further explore and address these issues and assist with coping strategies.

## How does the ONN support J.K. after surgery and at end of treatment?

J.K. has a residual 0.5 cm breast tumor. An axillary lymph node dissection is performed. Radiation is recommended to lower the risk of local recurrence.

Pregnancy after breast cancer is discussed by the medical oncologist with J.K. and her husband at the completion of treatment. Despite the fact that J.K. develops chemotherapy-induced amenorrhea, she understands that this does not mean she is infertile. In the same way, resuming her menses does not indicate that she is fertile. J.K. and her husband should seek future counsel with a fertility specialist and the medical oncologist if they try to conceive in the future. Pregnancy after treatment is possible and is not associated with a worse prognosis after breast cancer (de Pedro, Otero, & Martin, 2015).

J.K. also will be at increased risk for lymphedema. The ONN reinforces the education contained in the journey notebook. The ONN also schedules evaluations from a physical therapist and an occupational therapist immediately following J.K.'s surgery. The goal of these examinations will be to evaluate scar and tissue management, range of motion, posture, and potential subclinical symptoms for early intervention of lymphedema.

After a long emotional journey, tears are shed. J.K. verbalizes both the joy and fear commonly experienced at the end of treatment. The ONN offers continued support during this next phase of the journey—survivorship and wellness.

The ONN consults with J.K.'s physicians, who medically clear J.K. to participate in an evidence-based rehabilitation program at the cancer center. This supervised progressive training program provides education about lymphedema and helps build strength. J.K. is anxious to do what is within her control to promote wellness and prevent complications from lymphedema. She wants to feel comfortable and confident about maintaining a healthy and improved quality of life after cancer.

## Summary and Key Points

Young women with breast cancer are a unique patient population with complex needs. ONNs must be attentive to these needs. Facilitating early multidisciplinary care, education, advocacy, support, and assistance in identifying and achieving goals, ONNs play an important role in optimizing outcomes throughout the care continuum into survivorship. Increased knowledge and attention to the specific issues of young women with breast cancer can lower distress, improve satisfaction with decision making, and greatly influence quality of life—ultimately leading to positive long-term results for young women.

- Young women with breast cancer usually are defined as under age 40 and comprise 5%–7% of all women diagnosed (Reyna & Lee, 2014).
- Younger women usually present at more advanced stages, have more aggressive disease, and have lower rates of survival. This

makes treatment therapies physically and emotionally more burdensome (Greaney et al., 2015).

- Young women with breast cancer require careful attention and coordination by the ONN and the multidisciplinary team, as any treatments could affect their reproductive function.
- The potential health ramifications from cancer treatment can affect multiple body systems and have psychological effects (Adams et al., 2011).
- Fertility-related concerns are important to consider in all young women diagnosed with cancer.
- Many young patients diagnosed with cancer are unaware of fertility preservation options. An ONN can promote patient knowledge about fertility treatment options by advocating discussion with the care team.
- De Pedro et al. (2015) noted that 40%–50% of young women with breast cancer would like to become pregnant after treatment, yet studies show that only 4%–7% are able to conceive.
- The authors also found that less than 50% of women diagnosed under age 40 and only 10% of patients over the age of 40 will recover menses (de Pedro et al., 2015).
- The majority of women under the age of 35 resume menses within two years (National Comprehensive Cancer Network®, 2016). The risk of breast cancer recurrence in triple-negative disease peaks 2–3 years after surgery (Zhu, Perez, Hong, Li, & Xu, 2015).
- Providing information about advocacy organizations, such as Livestrong Fertility, Young Survival Coalition, and Living Beyond Breast Cancer, can offer additional knowledge and support (de Pedro et al., 2015).
- Younger women with breast cancer have greater psychosocial distress because they are suddenly faced with life changes such as fertility, body image, child care, menopause symptoms, sexual function, and career considerations.
- Potential recurrence, mortality, and the effect that breast cancer has on family can cause increased anxiety and fear in patients (Greaney et al., 2015).
- Connecting with support services, such as the Look Good Feel Better program; local resources for free wigs, hats, and scarves; nutrition programs; and other community and cancer center resources, is helpful for young adult patients.
- Online support groups and forums often appeal to young adult patients.

## Questions

### What resources regarding fertility are available to young women with breast cancer?

In addition to their healthcare team, the following are excellent resources for patients facing fertility issues (de Pedro et al., 2015):
- Reproductive medicine
- Livestrong Fertility
- Young Survival Coalition
- Living Beyond Breast Cancer

### What did the ONN do to help support J.K. and her husband?

The ONN guided J.K. and her husband through the cancer diagnosis by being present and addressing their concerns via education and support throughout the disease course. The ONN was instrumental in connecting J.K. with appropriate resources and validating her concerns and feelings regarding the influence of her breast cancer on her life (Greaney et al., 2015).

## References

Adams, E., McCann, L., Armes, J., Richardson, A., Stark, D., Watson, E., & Hubbard, G. (2011). The experiences, needs and concerns of younger women with breast cancer: A meta-ethnography. *Psycho-Oncology, 20,* 851–861. doi:10.1002/pon.1792

Davies, K.R., Cantor, S.B., & Brewster, A.M. (2015). Better contralateral breast cancer risk estimation and alternative options to contralateral prophylactic mastectomy. *International Journal of Women's Health, 7,* 181–187. doi:10.2147/IJWH.S52380

de Pedro, M., Otero, B., & Martin, B. (2015). Fertility preservation and breast cancer: A review. *Ecancermedicalscience, 9,* 503. doi:10.3332/ecancer.2015.503

Greaney, M.L., Sprunck-Harrild, K., Ruddy, K.J., Ligibel, J., Barry, W.T., Baker, E., ... Partridge, A.H. (2015). Study protocol for Young & Strong: A cluster randomized design to increase attention to unique issues faced by young women with newly diagnosed breast cancer. *BMC Public Health, 15,* 37. doi:10.1186/s12889-015-1346-9

National Cancer Institute. (2016). Genetics of breast and gynecologic cancers (PDQ®) [Health professional version]. Retrieved from http://www.cancer.gov/cancertopics/pdq/genetics/breast-and-ovarian/HealthProfessional/page2

National Comprehensive Cancer Network. (2016). *NCCN Clinical Practice Guidelines in Oncology (NCCN Guidelines®): Breast cancer* [v.2.2016]. Retrieved from http://www.nccn.org/professionals/physician_gls/pdf/breast.pdf

Reyna, C., & Lee, M.C. (2014). Breast cancer in young women: Special considerations in multidisciplinary care. *Journal of Multidisciplinary Healthcare, 7*, 419–429. doi:10.2147/JMDH.S49994

von Minckwitz, G., & Martin, M. (2012). Neoadjuvant treatments for triple-negative breast cancer (TNBC). *Annals of Oncology, 23*(Suppl. 6), vi35–vi39. doi:10.1093/annonc/mds193

Zhu, W., Perez, E.A., Hong, R., Li, Q., & Xu, B. (2015). Age-related disparity in immediate prognosis of patients with triple-negative breast cancer: A population-based study from SEER cancer registries. *PLOS ONE, 10*, e0128345. doi:10.1371/journal.pone.0128345

## CASE 8

# Developing a Relationship With a Newly Diagnosed Patient

Penny Daugherty, RN, MS, OCN®

J.T. is an unemployed 42-year-old woman with ovarian cancer. She decides to call the physician referral line at her local hospital because she can no longer breathe comfortably due to a grossly distended abdomen. She has watched two friends die from ovarian cancer—both terrifying experiences—and feels overcome with fear and profound grief concerning her own situation. J.T. also is experiencing intermittent periods of uncontrolled sobbing. The physician referral personnel know that any calls referring to gynecologic cancers are to be transferred immediately to the gynecologic oncology nurse navigator (ONN) for intake and management.

J.T. tells the ONN her symptoms, giving details between sobs. She reveals that she has no insurance and wonders about her ability to be treated at what she perceives to be an "upscale" community hospital. The ONN reassures J.T. that, because of the hospital's disparities program, she can be treated as she simultaneously applies for financial assistance (Cancer.Net, 2015). The ONN is concerned about J.T.'s reported distended abdomen and difficulty breathing and encourages her to come to the emergency department (ED) for evaluation.

The ONN stays late in the evening to personally welcome J.T. to the ED and to her room on the oncology unit, where she will be under the service of a gynecologic oncologist. The ONN assures J.T. that she is "in a safe place" and is going to receive excellent care. She also works with the radiology department and the gynecologic oncologist on-call to get a quick paracentesis. This is done for J.T.'s comfort and to procure any malignant cells that would establish a definitive diagnosis and enable the beginning of some type of treatment.

## What is the role of the ONN when working with patients with ovarian cancer?

Those who work with gynecologic oncology patients regularly observe that a sudden diagnosis of ovarian cancer can generate observable emotions of fear, dread, and panic for patients and their families. This is likely because of the cancer's dismal survival statistics. Many patients and families present in a highly distraught (occasionally hysterical) state, necessitating nursing and medical care similar to that given to a trauma patient (Benigno, 2013). Financial challenges can exacerbate the situation and add emotional barriers to logical thinking and the formation of a viable game plan regarding treatment options or choices. Patient-centered education is crucial to allay fears and reestablish a sense of control for the patient, not only at diagnosis, but also throughout the trajectory of care (Pedersen & Hack, 2010). The ONN must establish a sense of guidance, calm, and trust.

## How can the ONN help the patient?

When establishing a relationship with a newly diagnosed patient, it is crucial for the ONN to be available for all the patient's questions, concerns, and fears. As is the case with so many patients diagnosed with ovarian cancer, J.T. is in a crisis thought pattern. This posttraumatic stress disorder (PTSD)–type thinking will predominate and affect her reaction to everything that happens to her (National Cancer Institute [NCI], 2015). No correlation exists among level of education, ethnic background, and age when a patient is in a panic-stricken state; therefore, the ONN must proceed slowly and constantly assess the patient's ability to understand anything but brief and elementary constructs (Katz, 2012).

## How can the ONN help with the financial weight of a cancer diagnosis and treatment?

The ONN assists J.T. in obtaining financial assistance forms and encourages her to complete them as quickly as possible. J.T.'s sister proves a valuable support person, helping to complete forms with the hospital's disparities ONN to establish financial assistance. This relieves some stress for J.T., who has expressed humiliation in asking for financial help.

## What should the role of the ONN be in providing education?

Moving into the treatment phase, J.T. receives neoadjuvant chemotherapy. The patient's only prior orientation to chemotherapy was through an older aunt, who had become very nauseated and fatigued when in treatment; hence, the ONN's job now is to thoroughly educate J.T. about the new antiemetics and drugs and their possible side effects.

After a few educational sessions with her ONN, J.T. expresses a sense of preparedness and confidence. The ONN encourages her to call with any additional questions or concerns about the typical side effects associated with this type of treatment, such as peripheral neuropathy, nausea, fatigue, and taste and smell changes (American Cancer Society, 2013).

After J.T.'s debulking surgery (following her neoadjuvant chemotherapy), the ONN guides her toward beneficial nutritional choices and skin care. Chemotherapy and surgery can create skin dryness, sensitivity, and somatic alopecia.

The ONN also works with J.T. to reestablish a sense of physical and emotional awareness. When J.T. cries uncontrollably, the ONN guides her toward actions that create a sense of calm, including mindful meditation, relaxation breathing techniques, and journaling her experiences. J.T. tells the ONN that keeping a journal has become a daily, quiet joy for her, and she is thinking about taking a creative writing course at the local state college—something she never considered before her ovarian cancer diagnosis. Hoping to help other women with cancer, J.T. says that perhaps she can write about her journey in one of the periodicals that features personal stories from survivors of cancer.

## How did the ONN's relationship with J.T. evolve over time?

J.T. develops a sense of trust with her ONN. She calls when issues or questions surface, sharing many of her ongoing fears and apprehensions. The ONN becomes her sounding board and counselor during these times. Because of these conversations, the ONN also becomes equipped to guide J.T. through many anxiety-producing scenarios.

One of these scenarios is J.T.'s fear of resuming her sexual relationship with her husband. Her concerns center on her altered body image due to a long perpendicular scar that stretches from the pubis to above her navel. She also is not experiencing the sensations of arousal because of her chemotherapy-induced fatigue and altered sense of smell. The ONN is able to provide a "safe-space" atmosphere, offering suggestions for negligees to help J.T. with her body image and aromatherapy for her scent issues. The ONN also gives J.T. helpful NCI booklets concerning women's sexuality issues (Benigno, 2013).

J.T. tells the ONN that their relationship gives her a sense of "shelter" and self-empowerment that she cannot achieve with anyone else, especially her family. She says that some thoughts are "just too private to share." J.T. also verbalizes her feelings that her relationship with her ONN is unique, believing she can say or ask anything from her without feeling vulnerable (Shockney, 2010).

The ONN coordinates a support group at the local cancer support community. She encourages J.T. to join, believing she can find support and fellowship with other patients and their families. J.T. attends the support group and meets women with the same disease, forming friendships that will be very sustaining in the months and years that follow. The ONN also encourages J.T. to participate in walks at a local park, fashion shows put on by local boutiques, and activities sponsored by the Georgia Ovarian Cancer Alliance.

During the trajectory of her treatment, J.T. takes part in many of these offerings. She tells her ONN that she feels enveloped in the loving relationships that she has made along her journey. She says she no longer feels a sense of isolation and underlying dread, as she is able to meet and befriend other women who have been survivors for many years. This gives J.T. hope that she has a future after treatment.

## How can the ONN assist J.T. with her personal survivorship plan of care?

Between the initial rounds of neoadjuvant chemotherapy, the debulking surgery, six cycles of adjuvant chemotherapy, and six months of maintenance chemotherapy, J.T. has been in active treatment for over a year. During this time, she has planned her life around her treatments, laboratory tests, and support group activities. She confides to her ONN that her life has been totally altered by this experience. She believes she needs a new compass to pilot herself moving forward.

J.T. and her ONN have many conversations about the possibility of recurrence. J.T. understands this concept, as she has met women on their third or fourth treatment cycle. She says that recurrence is always on her mind; however, because of her relationship with her ONN and all the "gutsy" women she has met, J.T. is seeing her ovarian cancer diagnosis as an opportunity to reevaluate her life goals. She is now considering a change of career from being a realtor to pursuing education in social work. The ONN reinforces her availability as a sounding board and guide. J.T. says she feels uniquely nurtured through her ONN and all the women she has befriended. The fear that she felt at the beginning of her diagnosis has morphed into a "new sense of balance within herself." She has come to think of herself as a survivor.

To this date, J.T. has been disease free and is an active participant in support groups and survivorship activities. She speaks to medical students as a survivor and is a very vocal advocate for ovarian cancer fund-raising and awareness.

## Summary and Key Points

A diagnosis of ovarian cancer can cause patients to experience symptoms similar to PTSD and feel intense distress and anxiety for their family (NCI, 2015). It is essential that nurse navigation be initiated as quickly as possible—preferably at diagnosis—to establish trust and confidence in the navigator's ability to guide the patient through this sudden scenario, filled with incomprehensible and frightening vocabulary, treatments, and financial burden.

- The ONN must be able to provide a safe haven and act as a guide for patients.
- The ONN should be a translator for patients, as they may feel severely and emotionally challenged by the situation and the complexity of oncology treatment.
- Offering activities that will replace a sense of isolation and fearfulness is crucial to patients' mental health.

- Guiding patients toward other survivors is a valuable component in healing both mind and spirit.
- Recognizing that sexual issues can be profoundly disturbing, the ONN must be prepared to counsel patients and assist them in reestablishing a successful sense of intimacy with their partner.
- Understanding that ovarian cancer carries a significant possibility of recurrence, the ONN must help patients visualize themselves as survivors and assist them with a plan they are comfortable with moving forward (Lerner, 2015; Pedersen, Hack, McClement, & Taylor-Brown, 2014).

## Questions

### How important is sexual counseling to patients with ovarian cancer?

It is crucial to acknowledge the high probability of sexual side effects and create an open forum for patients to share their needs. This is a topic that ONNs should intently study. Written materials on the topic should be readily available for patients (Katz, 2012; Rathus, Nevid, & Fichner-Rathus, 2000).

### What is the role of ONNs in the psychosocial environment of patients?

ONNs have an opportunity to connect with their patients and assist them within the reality of their individual situations. Nurse navigation can support patients with factual and comprehensible discussions and guide them toward simplified choices. ONNs can normalize and validate the experiences of patients and help them prepare for future choices throughout their care and into survivorship (Lerner, 2015).

## References

American Cancer Society. (2013). *Sexuality for the woman with cancer: Cancer, sex, and sexuality.* Retrieved from http://www.cancer.org/acs/groups/cid/documents/webcontent/002912-pdf.pdf

Benigno, B.B. (2013). *The ultimate guide to ovarian cancer: Everything you need to know about diagnosis, treatment, and research.* Atlanta, GA: Sherryben Publishing House.

Cancer.Net. (2015). Introduction to the costs of cancer care. Retrieved from http://
www.cancer.net/navigating-cancer-care/financial-considerations/introduction
-costs-cancer-care

Katz, A. (2012). *After you ring the bell . . . 10 challenges for the cancer survivor.* Pittsburgh,
PA: Hygeia Media.

Lerner, M. (2015). Helping ourselves and others through a health crisis: Information, inspiration and hope. Retrieved from http://www.nationalcenterforemotio
nalwellness.org/#!health-crisis/z2xpx

National Cancer Institute. (2015). Cancer-related post-traumatic stress (PDQ®)
[Health professional version]. Retrieved from http://www.cancer.gov/about
-cancer/coping/survivorship/new-normal/ptsd-hp-pdq

Pedersen, A.E., & Hack, T.F. (2010). Pilots of oncology health care: A concept analysis
of the patient navigator role. *Oncology Nursing Forum, 37,* 55–60. doi:10.1188/10.
ONF.55-60

Pedersen, A., Hack, T.F., McClement, S.E., & Taylor-Brown, J. (2014). An exploration
of the patient navigator role: Perspectives of younger women with breast cancer.
*Oncology Nursing Forum, 41,* 77–88. doi:10.1188/14.ONF.77-88

Rathus, S.A., Nevid, J.S., & Fichner-Rathus, L. (2000). What is human sexuality? In S.
Rathus, J. Nevid, & L. Fichner-Rathus (Eds.), *Human sexuality in a world of diversity*
(4th ed., pp. 4–33). Boston, MA: Allyn and Bacon.

Shockney, L.D. (2010). Evolution of patient navigation. *Clinical Journal of Oncology
Nursing, 14,* 405–407. doi:10.1188/10.CJON.405-407

# CASE 9
# Cancer at a Young Age

Robin Atkinson, RN, BSN, OCN®

C.R. is a 26-year-old Caucasian woman who reports menorrhagia beginning prior to 2012. She is gravida 0, desires no children, and previously had taken oral contraceptives for one year. She denies having pelvic inflammatory disease or sexually transmitted infections. C.R.'s menstrual periods were "normal and light before the heavy bleeding started," and she has never had an abnormal Pap smear. She presents to her local emergency department (ED) with menorrhagia and critical hemoglobin of 5 g/dl. This pattern of abnormally heavy menstrual periods, along with additional episodes of heavy bleeding and hemoglobin in the 4–6 g/dl range, continues for several months.

C.R. is transferred from her local community hospital to the ED of a larger hospital connected to an accredited cancer center. She is admitted with a critical hemoglobin of 4.3 g/dl. C.R. is urgently evaluated by a gynecologic oncologist and taken to the operating room for examination under anesthesia. A biopsy reveals that C.R. has an invasive squamous cell carcinoma of the cervix. She has a staging positron-emission tomography–computed tomography (CT) that shows a prominent cervix/lower uterine segment with increased uptake and possible stage IIB cervical cancer.

Of note, C.R.'s admission weight is 288 pounds. Her oncology team recommends whole pelvic radiation and concurrent weekly cisplatin chemosensitization. C.R. is sent back to her local community for weekly cisplatin at 40 mg/m² and external beam radiation to the pelvis and periaortic lymph nodes. The healthcare team feels her compliance with treatment will be greater if she is treated in her local community versus requiring daily travel. Because parametrial involvement is suspected on examination, C.R. is not felt to be a good surgical candidate.

## How can a nurse navigator recognize the needs of a young patient with cervical cancer?

C.R. and her husband come back to the accredited cancer center for an internal radiation consult, as this type of radiation is not available in their community. C.R.'s home is more than three hours round-trip from the regional cancer center. She has a part-time job at a local pet superstore; however, because of her heavy menorrhagia, she will be unable to keep it.

At C.R.'s consult, the gynecologic oncology nurse navigator (ONN) recognizes C.R.'s immediate navigation problems of transportation longer than a three-hour commute and the cost of gasoline on a limited income.

During this meeting, the ONN uses age-appropriate interactions. Questions are directed to C.R. in a style of language she understands. Body image, self-care, and sexuality are almost always at the top of patients' list of questions. The ONN addresses each question, making sure C.R. has a clear understanding of each answer. The ONN also uses a distress screening tool, enabling her to ask more specific questions.

## How can the ONN help resolve barriers to care?

The ONN reviews services and possible assistance programs for C.R., such as those offered by the American Cancer Society, Cancer-Care, and State Employees Credit Union (SECU) Family House, as well as local funds to assist with medicine co-pays, gasoline, food, and payments for SECU housing. Arrangements are made for C.R. and one other person to come to the SECU housing the day before treatment begins, allowing her to rest and avoid early-morning travel.

## What barriers to care does the ONN identify?

The ONN identifies access to treatment as a barrier to care for C.R. Internal radiation treatment can be administered only at the regional cancer facility, which is three hours from C.R.'s home. At her local hospital, C.R. does have access to follow-up labs and an oncologist—if needed for immediate care—but does not have access to a gynecologic oncologist. Shalowitz, Vinograd, and Giuntoli (2015) found that patients with cervical cancer experienced better outcomes with gynecologic oncology care; however, the proximity of this care has caused barriers for C.R. and many women like her.

Approximately 14.8 million women in the United States (9.8% of the population) currently live in low-access counties (LACs) (Shalowitz et al., 2015). LACs are located more than 50 miles from a gynecologic oncologist. Women in these areas are more likely to be identified as Caucasian, Hispanic, American Indian, or Alaska Native. They typically have lower household incomes compared to women not living in LACs (Shalowitz et al., 2015).

Because of C.R.'s long travel time to the cancer center, arranging follow-up visits also presents a problem. As C.R.'s husband works, he has to rearrange his work schedule to drive her to radiation therapy. The couple worries that he may lose his job because of his increased number of schedule changes. C.R. realizes the importance of her treatment plan for a cure and has made every effort to plan ahead.

At the community cancer center, the ONN works with her care team to facilitate C.R.'s care to convenient times. Not only is access to care a barrier, but C.R. finds it difficult to pay for transportation. This problem is addressed by the ONN during their first meeting. C.R. is provided with assistance with travel costs through a fund for patients with low income, insurance gaps, and the everyday expenses of oncologic treatment.

Another barrier to care is C.R.'s employment status. The cancer center's resource specialist gives C.R. the local phone numbers and addresses to apply for Medicaid in her community. The ONN asks C.R. to call ahead for an appointment and inquire about documents needed for the application process. C.R. has the initiative and wants to take on her own responsibilities.

## How does the ONN follow C.R. through treatment?

The ONN closely follows C.R. throughout her treatment, offering emotional care and encouragement, education, and opportunities for C.R. and her family to ask questions at each visit and through weekly phone calls. Chaplain services are offered but declined by C.R. She comments that she does not need spiritual care, but she does appreciate the emotional support from her navigator. The ONN informs her about local gynecologic cancer wellness support group meetings, dates, and times. C.R. declines because of the long travel for a 90-minute meeting.

At the time of C.R.'s care, the cancer center does not employ a master of social work. A social worker is available as a patient advocate through a local agency, and the ONN gives C.R. contact information and also suggests other local resources. To maximize the benefits of her radiation treatment, dietitian services are offered to help support C.R.'s hemoglobin levels, which are constantly below 10 g/dl. This will promote adequate perfusion of tissues and decrease the possibility of anemia.

Throughout her radiation treatments, C.R. is assessed for nausea and vomiting, diarrhea, and skin issues. Her diarrhea is controlled by psyllium fiber (Lee et al., 2015). She has mild nausea during radiation and uses ondansetron hydrochloride for control. She also does this during chemotherapy. Overall, her hemoglobin returns to an acceptable range (11.6 g/dl) and her weight is reduced to 250 lbs (113.4 kg).

## What should the ONN's role be in assisting with a survivorship plan?

C.R.'s survivorship plan includes a one-on-one review with her ONN. When working with this young patient with cervical cancer, the ONN takes extra time to verbally discuss and give written information about follow-up care. The ONN and mid-level providers make every effort to involve the patient and—if C.R. allows it—her immediate family.

In general, communication is very important for this group. The ONN must consider the patient's social issues, romantic relationships, desire for independence, and career.

Follow-up care is every three months for C.R., which includes a Pap smear and pelvic examination for the first five years. Office visits alternate between radiation oncology and gynecologic oncology at the accredited cancer center.

C.R. also is assessed for issues with intercourse. She is educated on the use of a vaginal dilator to prevent vaginal stenosis and on vaginal lubrication to help with intercourse difficulties. Because C.R. and her husband have no desire to pursue a family, fertility-sparing measures are not indicated. C.R. is very clear regarding this desire in discussions with numerous physicians and healthcare professionals. CT scans are done for possible recurrent disease (National Comprehensive Cancer Network®, 2016).

## Summary and Key Points

C.R., a 26-year-old woman, originally presented to the ED with vaginal bleeding and a hemoglobin of 4.3 g/dl. She was diagnosed with stage IIB squamous cell carcinoma of the cervix at an accredited cancer center with a gynecologic oncologist and numerous radiation oncology specialists present. She was able to return to her community hospital with a medical oncologist specialist on staff for weekly cisplatin and external beam radiation to the pelvis and periaortic lymph nodes. Mild diarrhea was controlled with psyllium fiber and mild nausea with ondansetron hydrochloride. At the accredited regional cancer center, she was able to receive brachytherapy—five high-dose-rate tandem and ovoid insertions. ONN support maximized the availability of community resources to the patient.

Two years following treatment, C.R. receives normal Pap smears, pelvic examinations, and CT scans. She is expected to have a complete recovery.

In dealing with young patients with cervical cancer, ONNs can offer the following:

- Education on the long-term effects of radiation and chemotherapy
- Education on the use of vaginal dilators and lubricants
- Scheduling for follow-up maintenance visits for optimal care
- Information on survivorship clinics and nutritional consults
- Contact information for the healthcare team and advice on getting routine medical care with a primary care physician

## Questions

### Which groups of women are most likely to be affected by LACs?

All lower socioeconomic women of all backgrounds are likely to be affected. More than a third of the counties in the United States are located at least 50 miles from the nearest gynecologic oncologist. Approximately 15 million women have decreased access to gynecologic cancer care (Shalowitz et al., 2015).

## What is a major barrier to care addressed by ONNs?

Transportation to care is a major barrier addressed by ONNs (Payne, Jarrett, & Jeffs, 2008). Patients with cancer face many barriers and stressors, such as numerous patient visits, treatments, and tests. Because of these barriers, patients may forgo needed treatment.

## References

Lee, J., Cherwin, C., Czaplewski, L.M., Dabbour, R., Doumit, M., Duran, B., … Whiteside, S. (2016). Putting evidence into practice: Chemotherapy-induced nausea and vomiting. Retrieved from https://www.ons.org/practice-resources/pep/chemotherapy-induced-nausea-and-vomiting

National Comprehensive Cancer Network. (2016). *NCCN Clinical Practice Guidelines in Oncology (NCCN Guidelines®): Cervical cancer* [v.1.2016]. Retrieved from https://www.nccn.org/professionals/physician_gls/pdf/cervical.pdf

Payne, S., Jarrett, N., & Jeffs, D. (2008). The impact of travel on cancer patients' experiences of treatment: A literature review. *European Journal of Cancer Care, 9,* 197–213. doi:10.1046/j.1365-2354.2000.00225.x

Shalowitz, D.I., Vinograd, A.M., & Giuntoli, R.L., Jr. (2015). Geographic access to gynecologic cancer care in the United States. *Gynecologic Oncology, 138,* 115–120. doi:10.1016/j.ygyno.2015.04.025

# Rectal Cancer

Nicole Messier, RN, BSN, OCN®

H.F. is a 33-year-old woman with rectal cancer. She is married with two young sons and works full-time as an administrator at a local rehabilitation facility. She is a nonsmoker and reports occasional alcohol use (one to two drinks per month). Her paternal family history is negative for colorectal cancer, colitis, and polyps. Her maternal family history is unknown, as her mother was adopted; however, her mother does have irritable bowel disease (IBD).

H.F. developed some change in bowel habits as well as rectal bleeding approximately one year prior to her diagnosis. She was scheduled for a colonoscopy but found out she was pregnant with her second child; therefore, the colonoscopy was delayed. Throughout her pregnancy, she continued to have rectal bleeding with bright red blood per rectum, fecal urgency, and frequent bowel movements (8–12 times per day). Initially, these symptoms were considered to be the result of an inflammatory process, possibly IBD. After delivery, she was evaluated by a gastroenterologist, and a colonoscopy was performed. The colonoscopy revealed a 4 cm circumferential, friable mass around the lumen of the rectosigmoid junction. Biopsy of this mass was positive for an invasive, moderately differentiated adenocarcinoma.

## As recommended by evidence-based guidelines, what staging workup should H.F. have?

Following National Comprehensive Cancer Network® (NCCN®) guidelines, a carcinoembryonic antigen (CEA) test is obtained and found to be elevated at 14.8 ng/ml (Benson et al., 2012). H.F. undergoes staging with a computed tomography (CT) scan of the chest, abdomen, and pelvis. The CT scan reveals a circumferential, nonobstructing soft tissue mass involving the proximal rectum/rectosigmoid junction with prominent subcentimeter lymph nodes in the pelvis and retroperitoneum. No distant metastatic disease is identified.

A magnetic resonance imaging (MRI) of the pelvis is performed. A circumferential mass with multiple areas of extension into the muscularis propria is again identified. A few areas show 1–2 mm of extension beyond the muscularis propria, with one focus of invasion extending to the mesorectal fascia (MRF). Multiple lymph nodes measuring 5 mm and larger within and external to the MRF are present. Additionally, lymph nodes extending cranially along the inferior mesenteric vein are believed to contain metastatic disease. Locoregional MRI staging is reported as T3 MRF+, N2 (more than six lymph nodes suspected to harbor metastatic disease). H.F.'s clinical stage is documented as T3 N2a M0 (stage IIIB). Biopsy of the suspicious lymph nodes is not performed prior to initiation of therapy, as it is determined that biopsy results would not alter the recommended treatment plan.

## How does H.F.'s situation represent a multidisciplinary approach to cancer care?

H.F. is evaluated by a colorectal surgeon, who discusses her diagnosis as well as the standard of care for locally advanced rectal cancer. Treatment includes preoperative chemoradiation, followed by a low anterior resection with possible diverting loop ileostomy. She is referred by the surgeon to the gastrointestinal (GI) multidisciplinary clinic for evaluations with medical and radiation oncology.

After meeting with H.F. and reviewing her case, both the medical and radiation oncologists agree that preoperative chemoradiation is indicated; however, because of the extent of suspected nodal involvement on the MRI and the unclear correlation between lymphadenopathy and her postpartum status, it is decided that further evaluation with a positron-emission tomography (PET) scan is appropriate to properly stage the cancer.

H.F.'s PET scan shows increased radiotracer uptake within the rectal mass. An indeterminate to low level of increased radiotracer activity has been detected within the right deep pelvic lymph nodes and the small lymph nodes along the course of the inferior mesenteric vein. H.F.'s case is reviewed by the GI multidisciplinary conference tumor board. Because these high lymph nodes could possibly represent N3 disease, the board concludes that H.F. should initiate treatment with chemotherapy alone rather than chemoradiation. The rationale for this treatment is to initially avoid a major local therapy if a growing nonoperable distant disease exists. If appropriate, local therapy could be incorporated at a later date. H.F. also is encouraged to obtain a second opinion from another institution with medical and radiation oncology.

H.F.'s outside consultation yields two possible treatment options. The first includes giving the equivalent of 12 cycles of FOLFOX (folinic acid, 5-fluorouracil [5-FU], oxaliplatin), with restaging every four cycles. This is followed by chemoradiation, with radiation incorporated into the last six weeks of FOLFOX. Restaging and consideration for surgery would then occur.

A second option is to sandwich FOLFOX cycles around chemoradiation and surgery.

## What is the role of the GI nurse navigator in the multidisciplinary team?

The GI oncology nurse navigator (ONN) plays a pivotal part in the multidisciplinary team. "Nurse navigators work within the multidisciplinary cancer team as a patient advocate, care provider, educator, counselor, and facilitator" (Desimini et al., 2011, p. 26). ONNs effectively and efficiently facilitate key information between members of the multidisciplinary team and the patient. ONNs also are responsible for identifying patients for review at the multidisciplinary tumor board.

"Navigation of complex care becomes necessary when treatment recommendations may include chemotherapy, radiation, and surgery" (Case, 2011, p. 33). As part of the multidisciplinary team, the ONN acts as a consistent resource and point of contact for patients through treatment. This continuity helps strengthen a trusting relationship between the patient and ONN. It also allows the ONN opportunities to reassess ongoing patient needs and intervene as necessary.

## Based on H.F.'s diagnosis and treatment plan, how should the ONN communicate with her?

Gentry and Sellers (2014) noted that a key role of nurse navigation is to validate patients' understanding regarding diagnosis and proposed treatments. The authors stated that "understanding patients' needs and expectations is critical to ensure that appropriate information is provided for patients to effectively participate in informed treatment decision making" (p. 88). An ONN has the opportunity to empower a patient to take an active role in treatment decisions. A knowledgeable ONN can provide and reinforce necessary education about a diagnosis, clarify treatments plans, and answer any additional questions.

## What is H.F.'s treatment plan?

H.F. is treated with six cycles of neoadjuvant chemotherapy, including one cycle of capecitabine plus oxaliplatin (XELOX). This results in grade 4 enterotoxicity, requiring hospitalization.

This treatment is followed by five cycles of FOLFOX, which are very well tolerated at reduced doses. Follow-up imaging reveals an excellent response to chemotherapy from the primary tumor and lymph nodes.

After these cycles, H.F. undergoes bilateral oophoropexy to move her ovaries out of the pelvic radiation field. This is in an attempt to preserve ovarian function and avoid early menopause.

She next is treated with continuous-infusion 5-FU with radiation therapy to the pelvis and para-aortic lymph nodes. She receives two additional cycles of FOLFOX before proceeding with a low anterior resection and diverting loop ileostomy. Final pathology is ypT2, ypN0 (stage I).

H.F. asks the ONN, "I need to know that my team is all on the same page. Is it possible to have a group meeting with all of my doctors?"

One of Harold Freeman's core principles of patient navigation states, "There is a need to navigate patients across disconnected systems of care, such as primary care sites and tertiary care sites" (Freeman & Rodriguez, 2011, p. 3541). While it is quite common in multidisciplinary cancer clinics to coordinate same-day, same-location appointments, providers often consult with the patient separately. Providers' busy schedules simply may not allow the extra time that a multiprovider appointment could require. For many physicians, this is not a preferred scenario for patient visits.

Because of uncertainty with the extent of H.F.'s disease, open communication and active information sharing about her progress and the next steps of her treatment is imperative. Her case is formally reviewed multiple times at the GI multidisciplinary conference and informally among various members of the multidisciplinary team. H.F. is kept informed of thoughts and recommendations from all discussions. Her questions are answered by her physician team and reinforced by the GI nurse navigator to ensure understanding.

The GI nurse navigator acts as a consistent, reliable resource and advocates for the patient and her caregivers throughout the continuum of cancer care. The navigator also communicates directly with H.F.'s physicians to ensure seamless care during treatment.

H.F. sends a quick message to her treating physicians to schedule a group meeting, resulting in an informal discussion with her medical oncologist and surgeon. Both give H.F. the reassurance she needs, stating that her team is working together and openly communicating about her progress every step of the way.

## How can the ONN educate and guide H.F. with her personal survivorship plan of care?

The risk of pelvic recurrence is higher in patients with rectal cancer compared to those with colon cancer. Locally recurrent rectal cancer has frequently been associated with a poor prognosis (Benson et al., 2012); therefore, good surveillance and follow-up are indicated. Follow-up care usually consists of regular visits to the doctor's office for physical examinations, blood tests, and imaging studies. A colonoscopy is recommended one year after diagnosis of rectal cancer.

The GI nurse navigator should provide patient education regarding the need for adherence to surveillance appointments and tests to monitor for recurrence. Promotion of positive lifestyle changes, such as eating a healthy diet, maintaining a healthy weight, exercising, limiting alcohol, and quitting smoking, also is important to discuss with patients.

## Summary and Key Points

H.F. successfully completed neoadjuvant chemotherapy, chemoradiation, and surgery for stage III rectal cancer. She had good bowel function after ileostomy takedown, and initial follow-up CT scans revealed no evidence of metastatic disease. A colonoscopy one year after diagnosis was normal. H.F. is working full-time and enjoying her family and friends as she finds her "new normal" after her cancer diagnosis.

- NCCN develops and communicates scientific, evaluative information to better inform the decision-making process between patients and physicians, ultimately improving patient outcomes (NCCN, 2016).
- NCCN guidelines provide recommendations for the management of rectal cancer from clinical presentation through diagnosis, staging, treatment, surveillance, management of recurrent and metastatic disease, and survivorship.
- Colorectal cancer is the third most common cancer diagnosed in the United States in both men and women. According to the American Cancer Society (ACS), 39,610 new cases of rectal cancer were estimated in 2015, with about 9 out of 10 diagnosed in people older than age 50 (ACS, 2016a).
- Neoadjuvant treatment with chemotherapy and radiation therapy may shrink the cancer, often making surgery more effective for larger tumors and lowering the chance the cancer will come back in the pelvis (ACS, 2016b).
- The ONN communicates pertinent information and issues to the multidisciplinary team and the patient.
- The ONN serves as a patient advocate and liaison among specialties, identifying and removing barriers to comprehensive patient care across the cancer trajectory.

## Questions

### What is the role of the GI nurse navigator in the multidisciplinary team?

The GI nurse navigator plays a pivotal part in the multidisciplinary team. "Nurse navigators work within the multidisciplinary cancer team as a patient advocate, care provider, educator, counselor, and facilitator" (Desimini et al., 2011, p. 26).

## Why is communication important between the ONN and the patient?

Gentry and Sellers (2014) noted that a key role of nurse navigators is to validate a patient's understanding regarding the diagnosis and any proposed treatments. The authors stated that "understanding patients' needs and expectations is critical to ensuring that appropriate information is provided for patients to effectively participate in informed treatment decision making" (p. 88).

## References

American Cancer Society. (2016a). Key statistics for colorectal cancer. Retrieved from http://www.cancer.org/cancer/colonandrectumcancer/detailedguide/colorectal-cancer-key-statistics

American Cancer Society. (2016b). Treatment of rectal cancer, by stage. Retrieved from http://www.cancer.org/cancer/colonandrectumcancer/detailedguide/colorectal-cancer-treating-by-stage-rectum

Benson, A.B., III, Bekaii-Saab, T., Chan, E., Chen, Y., Choti, M.A., Cooper, H.S., ... Gregory, K.M. (2012). Rectal cancer. *Journal of the National Comprehensive Cancer Network, 10,* 1528–1564. Retrieved from http://www.jnccn.org/content/10/12/1528.full

Case, M.A.B. (2011). Oncology nurse navigator: Ensuring safe passage. *Clinical Journal of Oncology Nursing, 15,* 33–40. doi:10.1188/11.CJON.33-40

Desimini, E.M., Kennedy, J.A., Helsley, M.F., Denton, C., Rice, T.T., Stannard, B., ... Lewis, M.G. (2011). Making the case for nurse navigators—Benefits, outcomes, and return on investment. *Oncology Issues, 26*(5), 26–33. Retrieved from http://pages.nxtbook.com/nxtbooks/accc/oncologyissues_20110910/offline/accc_oncologyissues_20110910.pdf

Freeman, H.P., & Rodriguez, R.L. (2011). History and principles of patient navigation. *Cancer, 117*(Suppl. 15), 3539–3542. doi:10.1002/cncr.26262

Gentry, S.S., & Sellers, J.B. (2014). Navigation considerations when working with patients. In K.D. Blaseg, P. Daugherty, & K.A. Gamblin (Eds.), *Oncology nurse navigation: Delivering patient-centered care across the continuum* (pp. 71–120). Pittsburgh, PA: Oncology Nursing Society.

National Comprehensive Cancer Network. (2016). About NCCN. Retrieved from https://www.nccn.org/about/default.aspx

# CASE 11
# Lung Cancer

Kathleen A. Gamblin, RN, BSN, OCN®

M.V. is a 62-year-old woman who presents to her primary care physician complaining of a cough that has persisted for two weeks. After several courses of antibiotic treatment fail to resolve the cough, a chest x-ray is done, showing a suspicious area in M.V.'s right lung. She is referred to a pulmonologist, who is able to see M.V. the following week.

On examination and review of the chest x-ray, a computed tomography (CT) scan of the chest is ordered. The CT scan shows a mass in the right lung. The pulmonologist immediately orders a CT-guided biopsy. A thoracic oncology nurse navigator (ONN) is called. The patient is added to the next thoracic multidisciplinary clinic schedule for further workup and treatment planning.

## What should the thoracic ONN be aware of regarding a delayed diagnosis of lung cancer?

Variability in patient entry into the healthcare system can contribute to multifactorial delays in definitive diagnoses and treatment initiation (Blaseg, 2014). Patients may be treated for several months by their primary care physician for recurring pulmonary infections. Some patients may see a pulmonologist for diagnostic workup after an abnormal chest x-ray, while others may be sent directly to the hospital after being admitted for an oncologic emergency. Once in the healthcare system, patients often experience lengthy wait times, seeing up to four physician specialists, each with their own diagnostic testing criteria (Ellis & Vandermeer, 2011). This can lead to a more advanced stage at diagnosis, thus affecting the patient's prognosis. With emerging oncology nursing literature on the benefits of the thoracic ONN—particularly in the area of care coordination—it is vital to support and enhance these navigators' skills in proactively identifying patients, facilitating entry into the healthcare system, and coordinating timely care.

Prior to being seen at the thoracic multidisciplinary clinic, M.V. speaks with the thoracic ONN via telephone to collaboratively complete her medical history paperwork. Establishing this baseline enables the ONN to provide the physicians with additional information prior to seeing the patient. It also develops the relationship between the ONN and M.V. by determining M.V.'s current and potential needs through a navigation assessment.

## What is the importance of conducting a navigation assessment, and how often should it be done? Is a standardized assessment available?

Cancer is an unexpected life event. It becomes a part of daily life for patients and their families. Cancer does not lend itself to being set aside and ignored. It becomes a shadow that is always present. As patients and their families begin the cancer journey, they experience physical, emotional, social, psychological, spiritual, informational, and practical changes that can have a tremendous effect on their lives. Patients and their families may not have the ability to meet these changes; thus, their coping mechanisms may be compromised. Proactive assessment of these areas by the ONN can lead to the resources and assistance needed to decrease stress and anxiety for the patient and family.

No standardized assessment for navigation currently exists, but examples of assessments can be found online or in the Oncology Nursing Society's (ONS's) *Oncology Nurse Navigation: Delivering Patient-Centered Care Across the Continuum* (Blaseg, Daugherty, & Gamblin, 2014). As a specific example, the Northside Hospital Cancer Institute Oncology Patient Navigation Program created its navigation assessment based on the seven needs categories in Margaret Fitch's Supportive Care Framework for Cancer Care.

Currently, no guidance is available for how often navigation assessments should occur. The American College of Surgeons Commission on Cancer's (CoC's) standard (3.2) on psychosocial distress screening, which in some ways closely mirrors the navigation assessment, does not require assessment to be administered at a certain time but rather at a "pivotal medical visit" (American College of Surgeons, 2012, p. 77). This process requirement also would work well for navigation assessment.

Many ONNs currently complete a navigation assessment when they meet or speak with a patient for the first time. It is important to note that the needs of patients and their families are constantly changing as circumstances unfold. What may not be an issue when care begins may become an issue later, such as when a patient loses health insurance in the middle of treatment. It is advisable to identify key points within the navigation process to consistently reassess patients and their families.

M.V. and her husband are seen in the thoracic multidisciplinary clinic five days postbiopsy. She asks if the ONN would be willing to stay with them for the biopsy results. Within moments, M.V. is told she has small cell lung cancer. She and her husband appear visibly stunned by the news and simply nod when the pulmonologist explains that additional testing is needed to see how far the cancer has progressed. The pulmonologist politely exits the room after telling M.V. that several other physicians would be in to see her.

There is silence for a moment. Then, a barrage of questions spill from M.V. and her husband. The ONN gives basic answers at this point, promising to return after the physician visits to answer any additional questions and discuss the next steps.

## What is one of the primary roles of the ONN?

A primary role of the ONN is as an educator regarding the disease, treatment modalities, and available supportive care (Daugherty et al., 2014). Newly diagnosed patients and their families often will be overwhelmed and may have difficulty processing new information. "What did the physician tell you?" can be an extremely helpful open-ended question to determine what information patients and their families have absorbed. The ONN must be prepared to answer questions as many times as they are asked. It is important that patients and their families are able to reach the ONN in the days following diagnosis to ask these questions and clarify any information.

A question regarding level of education on a navigation assessment or medical history form can guide the ONN in gathering educational materials for patients. To ensure the best chance for comprehension, it is important that materials are tailored to each patient's education and literacy levels. A hospital library organizing patient materials by these levels will make it easier for the ONN to select literature best suited for each individual patient and family. Although educational materials for lung cancer range from pamphlets on understanding a pathology report to full books on survivorship, the ONN should only include the most pertinent materials to avoid overwhelming patients and their families.

After the physicians examine and speak with M.V., the ONN returns to answer additional questions. A basic educational packet about lung cancer is given to M.V. and her husband to read and review. M.V. verbalizes her fears of forgetting all the tests she needs, not knowing where to go for testing, and managing her transportation. Information is gathered regarding M.V.'s schedule. An appointment is set up for the following day to speak via telephone. Teaching sheets about various diagnostic tests and a map of the hospital campus are included in the educational packet.

The following day, the ONN notifies M.V. of all future diagnostic testing appointments, which are scheduled for her convenience. A calendar of appointments also is created and emailed to M.V. The teaching sheets included in the basic educational packet are reviewed. The ONN asks questions to clarify the patient's understanding of what is needed to prepare for each diagnostic test.

## What are the benefits of having both the ONN and patient involved in a multidisciplinary clinic setting?

Seek and Hogle (2007) described the development of a multidisciplinary thoracic cancer clinic and the thoracic ONN's role in the clinic. Prior to establishment of this clinic, diagnosis to treatment times for patients ranged from one to three months. This could have been attributed to the number of physicians the patient needs to see for diagnosis and treatment, to testing that is inadvertently repeated or needs to be repeated because of extended diagnostic time length, or to patients being confused or lost somewhere in the healthcare system.

By using an ONN in collaboration with physicians in patient care coordination, patients are scheduled for diagnostic testing and additional specialist appointments in an appropriate time-sensitive sequence (e.g., not scheduling a positron-emission tomography scan immediately after a lung biopsy). This fosters collaboration among all involved physicians (Daugherty et al., 2014).

ONNs can eliminate insurance issues by verifying that all preauthorizations and approvals have been received prior to testing. They also can cluster patient appointments to avoid multiple patient trips to the same testing facilities. ONNs are a valuable resource for any questions or concerns during the diagnostic process and can help patients who are easily confused or need extra assistance to complete diagnostic testing.

In response to the development of the thoracic multidisciplinary clinic described by Seek and Hogle (2007), 92% of patients initiated treatment within 14 days of clinic evaluation. Patient satisfaction with the clinic process was high, with an increase in the number of patients treated at the facility (Seek & Hogle, 2007). Other thoracic multidisciplinary clinics using thoracic ONNs also have reported significant improvements in the care timeline (Hunnibell, Slatore, & Ballard, 2013).

## What is the role of the ONN in educating the patient and family?

Once M.V.'s diagnostic testing is completed, it is determined that she has limited-stage small cell lung cancer. This news is conveyed on her return visit to the multidisciplinary clinic. M.V. and her husband agree to the recommended treatments.

The following day, the ONN receives a call from M.V.'s daughter, who lives in another state. The daughter states that she has done her "research on the Internet" and demands to know why her mother has not been given a "real" stage for her cancer. She believes the physicians "have no clue what they are doing" and wonders if the recommended treatments are "the right ones." She further voices her doubts about the physicians and treatment facility. After listening carefully to the daughter, the thoracic ONN asks open-ended questions and invites the daughter's feedback.

Afterward, the daughter states that she better understands the information given to her mother and is more comfortable with the treatment decisions.

## Why is the ONN's involvement with family and caregivers so important?

In the clinical setting, patients and their educational needs and decisions are the primary focus of the healthcare team. Although the patient remains the primary concern for the ONN, a strong emphasis also is placed on the patient's family and caregivers. ONS's *Oncology Nurse Navigator Core Competencies* consistently uses the wording "patient, family, and caregiver" in competencies centered on the communication process (ONS, 2013). Long-term illnesses such as cancer affect not only the patient but also family members, who often are put in the caretaker role. Family members also have the additional responsibility of coping with the patient's emotions along with their own (Bittman, Fast, Fisher, & Thomson, 2004; Van de Bovenkamp & Trappenburg, 2012). These emotions can be quite intense, especially during traditional milestones in the cancer continuum, when fear and apprehension are heightened (e.g., diagnosis, initiation of treatment, recurrence, end of life) (Pearson, 2006). The ultimate challenge can come when these intense emotions—most often manifesting as anger—are projected directly at the ONN. The ONN may feel personally attacked and withdraw or disengage from the family, caregiver, or even the patient (Pearson, 2006); however, Thomas (2003) noted that defensive behavior from the ONN is much more likely to result in anger. How the ONN responds will positively or negatively influence how these interactions continue. A facilitating communication style using open-ended questions and techniques of reflection, clarification, and empathy is the hallmark of a skilled nurse communicator (Pearson, 2006). This style will assist the ONN in developing strategies to assist the family, caregiver, and patient.

## How can the ONN engage the patient during active treatment?

M.V. goes on to receive her recommended treatments, calling the ONN with any related issues or questions. M.V. and her husband also request that the ONN attend physician appointments to help put new information into simpler terms. The ONN works with both M.V. and the medical oncology office to facilitate communication and ensure that all issues and potential problems are being communicated in a timely manner. The ONN also encourages M.V. and her husband to handle what issues they can on their own.

## What role does the ONN play in the multidisciplinary team?

ONNs often serve as the communication bridge between members of the multidisciplinary team. It is important that ONNs are seen as facilitators of communication instead of a barrier. Any information that an ONN receives regarding the patient's treatment and care should be directly communicated to the multidisciplinary team to avoid interference with the patient–physician relationship. It is preferable that patients, families, and caregivers communicate directly with the multidisciplinary team. If this becomes difficult, ONNs should assist with communication. ONNs should always work toward empowering patients, families, and caregivers.

## How can the ONN remain a resource after M.V. completes active treatment?

After a year of treatment—during which time there was a positive response to chemotherapy—M.V. begins to complain of headaches. A magnetic resonance imaging (MRI) scan of her brain is ordered. Several brain lesions are found. Despite her physician's belief that she would benefit from further treatment, M.V. and her family make the difficult decision to decline treatment and seek palliative care. Secondary to the physician's referral and the ONN's recommendation, M.V. seeks hospice care and dies peacefully in her home, surrounded by her husband and children.

## How can the ONN assist patients and families in transitioning to palliative care?

When reaching the acknowledged end-of-life stage, a unique dilemma may present in which patients, families, and caregivers rely heavily on their ONN and do not wish to transition to other care providers. This relationship, which may help to remove patient barriers along the journey, may in itself become a barrier to patients receiving end-of-life resources. By promoting the work of the hospice team, the ONN can reassure patients, families, and caregivers that they will receive the same level of resources and support as before. Any questions and concerns should be directed to the hospice team. This establishes clear boundaries and prevents duplication of services and role confusion (Blaseg, 2014).

## Summary and Key Points

The journey of a patient with lung cancer can be particularly challenging. Unlike most other cancers, this journey is often marked with advanced disease at diagnosis, a low five-year survival rate, and a higher mortality rate. Using an ONN in the diagnostic process to coordinate care can be instrumental in decreasing the time between suspicious findings and the diagnosis or between the diagnosis and treatment. Beyond the patient's physical symptoms and clinical state, many other issues exist, including financial, educational, social, transportation, housing, and varied emotional reactions to the diagnosis. Conducting a thorough assessment of needs close to the first meeting or introduction to the patient is important to highlight issues. The navigation assessment should continue at pivotal points throughout the cancer continuum, as new issues may present. Some organizations may choose to combine the navigation assessment into a distress screening tool, allowing both navigation and other disciplines to be alerted to potential issues and barriers for the patient.

Patients and caregivers need education around the disease process, including testing and treatments needed and support services available. Before providing any educational material, a health literacy assessment or a query as to the patient's educational level can assist the ONN in determining the most helpful educational materials. All educational materials should be tailored to meet patient and caregiver health literacy levels, comprehension, and needs. Although the ONN's primary responsibility remains to the patient, special attention also should be paid to the caregiver and family. The ONN can be pivotal in helping caregivers and families understand what is happening and what will occur next in the continuum of care. The relationship between the ONN and the patient and caregiver is a strong one. When end-of-life issues arise, a level of trust allows the ONN to assist the family in transitioning to hospice care.

- The ONN's involvement can contribute to a decreased time from a suspicious finding to a definitive diagnosis. Earlier diagnosis can result in earlier cancer staging, leading to better outcomes.

- A navigation assessment should be repeated at pivotal points along the cancer continuum, as patient and caregiver needs change over time.

- As a primary task of the ONN, education should include a health literacy assessment on an individual basis. It should be tailored to the patient and caregivers and be supported by an easily accessible ONN.

- The ONN serves as a resource for patients, families, and caregivers; however, the ONN should maintain the patient's privacy at all times.

- The ONN should function as a liaison for effective communication throughout the multidisciplinary team, empowering patients to communicate with team members.

- The ONN should not disengage when active treatment is completed or stopped, as he or she can offer helpful patient resources on palliative care, hospice, or survivorship.

## Questions

### What factors put M.V. at risk for small cell lung cancer?

M.V. reported on her intake questionnaire for the clinic that she had a 50-pack-year history of smoking. Pack-years are determined by multiplying the number of packs per day by the number of years smoked (National Cancer Institute, n.d.). Tobacco smoke, either by primary inhalation or secondary exposure, is the leading cause of small cell lung cancer. Smokers exposed to radon or asbestos are at an even higher risk (American Cancer Society, 2015).

### What is the duration of the ONN's time with the patient?

With first introductions, expectations should be given as to how long the ONN will journey with the patient (Freeman & Rodriguez, 2011). The ONN's job description, which details role responsibilities, sets clear boundaries and allows for the transition of the patient to the next navigator or healthcare provider along the continuum (Blaseg, 2014).

## References

American Cancer Society. (2016). Lung cancer (non-small cell). Retrieved from http://www.cancer.org/acs/groups/cid/documents/webcontent/003115-pdf.pdf

American College of Surgeons. (2012). *Cancer program standards 2012: Ensuring patient-centered care* [v1.2.1]. Retrieved from https://www.facs.org/~/media/files/quality%20programs/cancer/coc/programstandards2012.ashx

Bittman, M., Fast, J.E., Fisher, K., & Thomson, C. (2004). Making the invisible visible: The life and time(s) of informal caregivers. In N. Folbre & M. Bittman (Eds.), *Family time: The social organization of care* (pp. 69–89). New York, NY: Routledge.

Blaseg, K.D. (2014). Getting started as a nurse navigator. In K.D. Blaseg, P. Daugherty, & K.A. Gamblin (Eds.), *Oncology nurse navigation: Delivering patient-centered care across the continuum* (pp. 15–42). Pittsburgh, PA: Oncology Nursing Society.

Blaseg, K.D., Daugherty, P., & Gamblin, K.A. (Eds.). (2014). *Oncology nurse navigation: Delivering patient-centered care across the continuum.* Pittsburgh, PA: Oncology Nursing Society.

Daugherty, P., Messier, N.G., dela Rama, F., Stern, H., Keen, S.J., & Blaseg, K.D. (2014). Cancer site-specific navigation. In K.D. Blaseg, P. Daugherty, & K.A. Gamblin (Eds.), *Oncology nurse navigation: Delivering patient-centered care across the continuum* (pp. 137–174). Pittsburgh, PA: Oncology Nursing Society.

Ellis, P.M., & Vandermeer, R. (2011). Delays in the diagnosis of lung cancer. *Journal of Thoracic Disease, 3,* 183–188. doi:10.3978/j.issn.2072-1439.2011.01.01

Freeman, H.P., & Rodriguez, R.L. (2011). History and principles of patient navigation. *Cancer, 117*(Suppl. 15), 3537–3540. doi:10.1002/cncr.26262

Hunnibell, L.S., Slatore, C.G., & Ballard, E.A. (2013). Foundations for lung nodule management for nurse navigators. *Clinical Journal of Oncology Nursing, 17,* 525–531. doi:10.1188/13.CJON.525-531

National Cancer Institute. (n.d.). *NCI dictionary of cancer terms.* Retrieved from http://www.cancer.gov/publications/dictionaries/cancer-terms?cdrid=306510

Oncology Nursing Society. (2013). *Oncology nurse navigator core competencies.* Retrieved from https://www.ons.org/sites/default/files/ONNCompetencies_rev.pdf

Pearson, K. (2006). Interpersonal and therapeutic skills inherent in oncology nursing. In R.M. Carroll-Johnson, L.M. Gorman, & N.J. Bush (Eds.), *Psychosocial nursing care along the cancer continuum* (2nd ed., pp. 385–401). Pittsburgh, PA: Oncology Nursing Society.

Seek, A.J., & Hogle, W.P. (2007). Modeling a better way: Navigating the healthcare system for patients with lung cancer. *Clinical Journal of Oncology Nursing, 11,* 81–85. doi:10.1188/07.CJON.81-85

Thomas, S.P. (2003). Anger: The mismanaged emotion. *MEDSURG Nursing, 12,* 103–110.

Van de Bovenkamp, H.M., & Trappenburg, M.J. (2012). Comparative review of family–professional communication: What mental health care can learn from oncology and nursing home care. *International Journal of Mental Health Nursing, 11,* 366–385. doi:10.1111/j.1447-0349.2011.00798.x

# CASE 12
# Genitourinary Cancer

Lori McMullen, RN, MSN, OCN®

C.R. is a 50-year-old man with no significant medical history who originally reported one month of painless, bloody urine. A urinalysis indicates red blood cell/high power field greater than 50 (0–2 = normal limit [NL]) and white blood cell at 20 (0–5 = NL). An ultrasound of his bladder shows a filling deficit. A cystoscopy reveals a left lateral wall bladder tumor covering the ureteral orifice. A transurethral resection of the bladder tumor (TURBT) shows a high-grade papillary urothelial carcinoma with infiltration of the lamina propria. A repeat TURBT one month later confirms a diagnosis of stage T1 bladder cancer.

## What should an oncology nurse navigator (ONN) know about bladder cancer?

C.R.'s hematuria is a classic presentation of bladder cancer. Additional symptoms may include dysuria, burning, frequency, and pelvic pain (Maliski, 2016). Bladder cancer is the fourth most common cancer in the United States and the eighth most common cause of cancer death. Men are four times more likely than women to be affected by bladder cancer, with a median age of 65 at diagnosis. The greatest risk factor associated with bladder cancer is tobacco use; C.R. has a 20-pack-year smoking history. Other risk factors include exposure to chemicals used in textiles, dyes, rubbers, and leathers; cyclic chemicals (benzenes and arylamines); use of pioglitazone hydrochloride; arsenic in well water; chronic bladder infection; and exposure to chemotherapy with cyclophosphamide, which also is recognized as possibly contributing to the development of the disease (American Cancer Society

[ACS], 2016; Cancer.Net, 2015; Maliski, 2016). Diagnostic testing may include a TURBT to collect biopsy samples. A positive biopsy will lead to additional testing to determine the stage or if the cancer has spread to other organs. Testing may include IV pyelography, computed tomography (CT) scan, or magnetic resonance imaging (MRI) (ACS, 2016). Bladder cancer has four major classifications: urothelial carcinoma (95% of cases), squamous cell carcinoma (1%–2%), adenocarcinoma (1%), and small cell tumors (1%). Within these classifications, the tumor is graded using consensus criteria established by the World Health Organization and the International Society of Urological Pathology. It is staged using the American Joint Committee on Cancer staging system (Maliski, 2016).

## How can the ONN assist the patient in understanding treatment options?

Management of bladder cancer focuses on preserving bladder function and preventing progression of the disease. Treatment options are presented to C.R. from the National Comprehensive Cancer Network® guidelines, which include TURBT to remove the tumor, intravesicular therapy, radical cystectomy with bladder diversion, systemic chemotherapy, radiation therapy, and concurrent chemotherapy with radiation therapy. C.R. is offered intravesicular bacillus Calmette-Guérin (BCG) for treatment of his T1 bladder cancer (Barlow & Shepard, 2014).

## How can the ONN assist C.R. during the trajectory of his disease?

Two years later, C.R. develops abdominal pain. CT scans of the abdomen and pelvis show extensive retroperitoneal and internal right iliac node enlargement with surrounding inflammation. New nodular prominence of the right adrenal gland also is noted. The patient undergoes a CT-guided biopsy of a right iliac node. Pathology confirms malignant cells consistent with urothelial primary. A positron-emission tomography scan shows hypermetabolic areas in the retroperitoneum, pelvis, right hilum, lower neck, lungs, and bilateral adrenals. C.R.'s cancer has advanced to stage IV. He is offered MVAC (methotrexate, vinblastine, doxorubicin, cisplatinum) chemotherapy every two weeks (accelerated) with granulocyte–colony-stimulating factor (G-CSF). C.R.'s medical oncologist asks him to make an appointment with an ONN.

The ONN refers to the patient's chart to confirm the anticipated start date for treatment and the prescribed chemotherapy regimen with G-CSF. The ONN should determine what C.R. understands about his diagnosis and the chemotherapy regimen prescribed by the medical oncologist. The ONN is aware that the five-year survival rate for stage IV bladder cancer is 15% (ACS, 2016).

When the ONN meets with the patient, C.R. is very tearful and upset with his diagnosis and prognosis. The ONN offers emotional support. Because no social worker exists at the cancer center, the ONN refers the patient to a Cancer *Care* oncology social worker, which C.R. accepts. The ONN also refers the patient to the Bladder Cancer Advocacy Network (www.bcan.org), an online support and education resource, and to written information from ACS and Cancer .Net.

## What is the ONN's role in educating the patient?

C.R. expresses anxiety about starting systemic chemotherapy. The ONN encourages him to review the chemotherapy regimen and its possible side effects. Typical side effects of MVAC include anemia, thrombocytopenia, neutropenia, fatigue, weight gain or loss, hair loss, sore mouth, altered taste, and constipation (Cancer .Net, 2015). Additionally, doxorubicin may cause heart damage and red urine. C.R. also will need to be educated about the signs and symptoms of neuropathy. The ONN reinforces the importance of G-CSF.

## What further questions should the ONN ask?

The ONN reviews the patient's social situation to assess for potential or real barriers to care. C.R. is divorced and has custody of his 11-year-old daughter. They live in a single family home. His sister lives nearby and cares for their older adult parents. His brother lives in Florida.

C.R. carries healthcare benefits covering 90% of his medical bills. He drinks alcohol socially and is 20 pounds overweight. Although he had stopped smoking at the time of his initial diagnosis, he admits to smoking half a pack of cigarettes a day. He works for a large company and used to be out of the country for months at a time. After his diagnosis, his employer adjusted C.R.'s role to allow him to stay in the United States to receive treatment. With a diagnosis of metastatic disease, C.R. will opt for short-term disability. The ONN encourages C.R. to look into the Family and Medical Leave Act (FMLA) to protect his position with his company.

C.R. has received four of six planned cycles of MVAC chemotherapy when he complains of increasingly painful tingling and numbness in his hands and feet, affecting his ability to walk and perform activities of daily living.

## What can the ONN ask the patient to assess for peripheral neuropathy?

Chemotherapy-induced peripheral neuropathy affects 64%–85% of patients who receive neurotoxic chemotherapy (e.g., taxanes, platinum-based agents, vinca alkaloids, thalidomide, bortezomib) (Tofthagen & Irwin, 2014). The ONN should assess physical function, such as gait disturbance; the ability to button buttons, tie shoes, or hold utensils to eat and cook; and the presence of numbness, burning, itching, dizziness, and weakness (Maxwell, 2013). C.R.'s ONN asks him to pick up coins from a flat surface; he struggles and is unsuccessful. C.R. is diagnosed with grade 2 peripheral sensory and motor neuropathy (National Cancer Institute, 2010) and treated with oxycodone for a pain level of 8 out of 10. He also receives physical therapy for the resulting gait disturbance.

Four months into treatment, C.R. continues on oxycodone and is tearful whenever he meets with the ONN. "I am not sure what the future will bring," he says. He complains of poor memory, weakness, and fatigue.

A psychosocial distress tool is administered. This standard was adopted by the hospital's cancer center in 2015. It is mandated by the American College of Surgeons Commission on Cancer.

This step triggers a social worker referral, which C.R. refuses. He complains, "She did not help me much the last time. My oncologist has prescribed paroxetine."

The ONN suggests a conversation with the mental health nurse practitioner; C.R. accepts. The ONN facilitates the appointment after speaking with the oncologist. C.R. is diagnosed with depression related to a chronic illness and is scheduled for routine visits with the nurse practitioner. C.R. shares that he is no longer able to perform his job, has applied for Social Security Disability Insurance (SSDI), and will have no medical insurance coverage at the end of the month. He remarks, "I don't know how I am going to be able to provide for my daughter and pay for my care. My life is falling apart. I may have to move to Florida to stay with my brother. Who is going to take care of my cancer there? I don't have a doctor in Florida!"

## How can the ONN help C.R. manage his evolving obstacles?

The ONN refers C.R. to a financial counselor at her institution. The ONN also investigates possible options for pharmaceutical assistance programs and local and national financial assistance charities.

Following his meeting with the financial counselor, C.R. reports to the ONN that he qualifies for state charity care at 100%. He is responsible for finding coverage through the insurance marketplace (Patient Protection and Affordable Care Act [ACA]) when enrollment opens. The ONN offers to explore options for cancer treatment in Florida.

## Summary and Key Points

A 50-year-old man with stage IV bladder cancer experienced physical, social, and emotional complications from his cancer and chemotherapy treatment. After four cycles of treatment, he experienced grade 2 peripheral neuropathy, which caused constant pain and affected his overall ability to walk, perform activities of daily living, and work. Losing his job resulted in loss of income and medical insurance. It is probable that metastasis of his disease, the onset of peripheral neuropathy from the treatment, and the loss of his job contributed to his diagnosis of depression. The ONN influenced the care of this patient through education, emotional support, referrals to collaborating support services, and assistance with continuity of care by locating a medical oncologist in Florida.

- BCG is immunotherapy that uses the body's immune system to attack cancer cells (Society of Urologic Nurses and Associates, 2013).
- BCG is a bacterium related to tuberculosis. Patients must be informed that they will always have a positive purified protein derivative (PPD) skin test after receiving BCG (Barlow & Shepard, 2014).
- BCG is instilled directly into the bladder via a catheter and released after two hours via voiding (Barlow & Shepard, 2014).
- Proper fluid intake is imperative with cisplatin. Instruct patients to drink at least two to three quarts of fluid every 24 hours and to report absence of urine output in 12 hours.
- Neutropenia is a concern for accelerated MVAC. A fever of 100.4°F (38°C) or chills without fever should be reported immediately. The patient will need a working thermometer and instructions on how to contact the medical oncologist after hours.
- SSDI is paid when eligible patients can demonstrate that they can no longer work because of a medical condition expected to last at least one year or result in death. Processing an application can take up to five months. Medicare coverage is available after two years of receiving disability benefits (Social Security Administration, 2015).
- The ACA, first available in 2013, offers medical insurance for purchase from a state marketplace or exchange. Plans are competitively priced with a cap on what consumers must pay for out-of-pocket costs. Financial assistance in the form of cost-sharing and reduced monthly payments is available based on income level and family size (Cancer and Careers, 2014).
- Lifestyle modification should be addressed as a part of treatment. If needed, patients should be referred to a smoking cessation program and a registered dietitian for help with making healthy food choices.
- Short-term disability, managed by an employer or home state, typically lasts up to six months, covers 26 weeks away from work, and pays between 55% and 100% of wages (Cancer and Careers, 2014).
- For eligible employees, FMLA guarantees protection of health insurance benefits, unpaid leave, and the ability to return to a previous job position (or equivalent job with same salary) for a period of up to 12 weeks in a 12-month period (U.S. Department of Labor, n.d.).
- Generally, patients recall only 25% of medical information delivered verbally. Ensure that patients receive written information

concerning their chemotherapy regimen and the possible side effects (Sandberg, Sharma, & Sandberg, 2012).

## Questions

### When educating patients with bladder cancer, what should the ONN include concerning the use of BCG?

BCG helps prevent cancer from recurring in the bladder lining. It also reduces the risk of it becoming invasive. BCG bacterium is related to tuberculosis. These patients will always have a positive PPD for tuberculosis. Because BCG is a live virus, patients should be taught to avoid urine splash on toilet seats and exposure on body parts (Barlow & Shepard, 2014).

### What resources can the ONN provide regarding employment and insurance concerns?

The ONN can refer patients to the financial advocate at a cancer center as well as their employer's human resources department to discuss FMLA, short-term disability, the Consolidated Omnibus Budget Reconciliation Act, and other options (Cancer and Careers, 2014; Social Security Administration, 2015).

## References

American Cancer Society. (2016). Bladder cancer. Retrieved from http://www.cancer.org/acs/groups/cid/documents/webcontent/003085-pdf.pdf

Barlow, W., & Shepard, L.H. (2014). Care of the patient with bladder cancer. *Nursing Made Incredibly Easy!, 12*, 40–48. doi:10.1097/01.NME.0000452685.17977.66

Cancer and Careers. (2014). *Living and working with cancer workbook.* Retrieved from http://www.cancerandcareers.org/grid/publication/pdf/4d6bc32623380f5753000037/publication_pdf.1423597756.Living___Working_with_Cancer_Workbook_4th_Ed.pdf

Cancer.Net. (2015). Bladder cancer—overview. Retrieved from http://www.cancer.net/cancer-types/bladder-cancer/view-all

Maliski, S.L. (2016). Cancers of the urinary system. In J.K. Itano (Ed.), *Core curriculum for oncology nursing* (5th ed., pp. 117–131). St. Louis, MO: Elsevier.

Maxwell, C. (2013). Quality-of-life considerations with taxane-based therapy in metastatic breast cancer. *Clinical Journal of Oncology Nursing, 17*(Suppl. 1), 35–40. doi:10.1188/13.CJON.S1.35-40

National Cancer Institute Cancer Therapy Evaluation Program. (2010). *Common terminology criteria for adverse events* [v.4.03]. Retrieved from http://evs.nci.nih.gov/ftp1/CTCAE/CTCAE_4.03_2010-06-14_QuickReference_8.5x11.pdf

Sandberg, E.H., Sharma, R., & Sandberg, W.S. (2012). Deficits in retention for verbally presented medical information. *Anesthesiology, 117,* 772–779. doi:10.1097/ALN.0b013e31826a4b02

Social Security Administration. (2015). Disability benefits. Retrieved from https://www.ssa.gov/pubs/EN-05-10029.pdf

Society of Urologic Nurses and Associates. (2013). Bladder cancer patient fact sheet. Retrieved from https://www.suna.org/download/members/bladderCancer.pdf

Tofthagen, C., & Irwin, M. (2014). Peripheral neuropathy. In M. Irwin & L.A. Johnson (Eds.), *Putting evidence into practice: A pocket guide to cancer symptom management* (pp. 201–210). Pittsburgh, PA: Oncology Nursing Society.

U.S. Department of Labor. (n.d.). *Need time? The employee's guide to the Family and Medical Leave Act.* Retrieved from http://www.dol.gov/whd/fmla/employeeguide.pdf

# Advanced Prostate Cancer

Frank dela Rama, RN, MS, AOCNS®, AGN-BC

R.M. is a 77-year-old man with prostate cancer. He was diagnosed by a local urologist, but not one who routinely provides referrals for prostate cancer navigation. While doing a general search online for prostate cancer resources in the area, R.M.'s daughter discovers a nurse navigator who should be able to help her father. After getting a few details over the phone, the navigator believes that R.M.'s prostate cancer sounds like late-stage disease. The navigator spends more than 30 minutes addressing all of the daughter's questions during the call, including the following:

- Why not surgery?
- Why not radiation?
- Why only hormones?
- Why did it take so long to check R.M.'s prostate-specific antigen (PSA)?
- How long does my father have to live?

The patient's daughter had not been at the initial consult and has only secondhand information from her parents. She does know that her father's Gleason score is 4 + 5 and his PSA is a little over 10 ng/ml. Given that her father is already in his late 70s with other comorbidities, including cardiac and renal disease, surgery is not a good option. In reviewing the National Comprehensive Cancer Network® (NCCN®) guidelines, the navigator notes that an option to consider is radiation with or without hormone treatment. R.M.'s urologist initiates the hormone treatment, but a radiation oncology consult is not ordered.

With multiple questions and too many unknowns, the navigator invites the family for an office visit. The navigator also reaches out to the patient's urologist and primary care provider to gather more information to support the family in making treatment decisions.

## Based on past medical history and a possible treatment plan, how should the nurse navigator communicate with R.M.?

In prostate cancer, navigators often are first connected with patients and families facing a new diagnosis. This may present as a localized, low- to intermediate-risk disease or perhaps as an advanced, high-risk disease (Daugherty et al., 2014). NCCN guidelines assist healthcare providers in determining the proper course of care (specific to risk level) and other clinical aspects. Yet, even within one particular risk cohort, multiple treatment options are available (NCCN, 2016). These options all may be equally effective, adding difficulty to the decision-making process for treatment for the patient, his family, and the healthcare team.

Providing patient education on treatment guidelines and facilitating shared decision making are key tasks specific to the prostate cancer nurse navigator role.

## What are the possible treatment options for R.M.?

R.M. and his wife and daughter all meet with the navigator. Since the first call with his daughter, the navigator has connected with R.M.'s urologist and primary care provider to get a better sense of the situation. Without any symptoms, the plan is to reserve radiation until it is needed, which is reasonable given R.M.'s clinical picture (T2a, Gleason 9 with 7 cores positive, PSA 10.2 ng/ml) and no reported back pain.

Using NCCN guidelines (2016), the navigator can first determine all possible treatment options, explaining the benefits and risks related to each option to the patient and his family. To initially stratify risk, the NCCN guidelines start with T stage, Gleason score/pathology, and PSA level. R.M. has a low-risk T stage (T2a), an intermediate-risk PSA level (between 10–20 ng/ml), but a very high-risk pathology finding (> 4 cores with Gleason score 8–10). Treatment options would include the following (NCCN, 2016):

- External beam radiotherapy (EBRT) + androgen deprivation therapy (ADT) × 2–3 years
- EBRT + brachytherapy ± ADT × 2–3 years
- Radical prostatectomy + pelvic lymph node dissection

R.M.'s daughter initially asked about all these options by phone, so her concerns are valid given what she knows. With a PSA level greater than 10 ng/ml, a bone scan needs to be performed. A computed tomography (CT) scan of the abdomen and pelvis also is ordered. During their second visit, the navigator reviews these results, which unfortunately show lymph node involvement on the CT, yet no metastases on the bone scan. R.M. still reports minimal to no pain.

With the staging now upgraded to T2a N1 M0, NCCN treatment options change from very high risk to metastatic disease in the regional lymph nodes:
- ADT
- EBRT + ADT × 2–3 years

## How can the navigator help R.M. weigh these options?

At this point, the shared decision-making process should take into consideration concrete clinical aspects and other less measureable (but crucial) aspects, such as possible side effects, effect on quality of life, and patient preferences. A variety of shared decision-making tools exist to help navigators work with patients in treatment (Ottawa Hospital Research Institute, 2015; Palo Alto Medical Foundation, 2010).

After completing the prostate cancer treatment decision-making tool (Palo Alto Medical Foundation, 2010), it is determined that R.M.'s priorities are centered on maintaining quality of life and avoiding treatment side effects entirely, as opposed to getting the cancer out or pursuing any aggressive or experimental treatment methods. ADT alone was the treatment of choice, reserving EBRT if R.M. becomes more symptomatic.

At his third visit, R.M. is not having any problems with the regimen of bicalutamide and leuprolide acetate, which he started about one month earlier; however, he does have occasional mild hot flashes. There is plenty of worry in the room. R.M. and his wife are from an "old school" generation—one that obeys doctor's orders and does not want to disappoint the esteemed professionals providing R.M.'s care.

R.M.'s daughter is a bit more inquisitive, but she also is having difficulties with the role reversal of caring for her father. On top of this, R.M. is a stoic man, not inclined to disclose many symptoms.

Not wanting to burden his family, he hopes to power through treatment as a lone warrior.

After a series of questions, R.M. and his family eventually become more comfortable with the plan for managing advanced prostate cancer. While not truly curable, it definitely is treatable for a long period of time. In the interim, they complete consultations with the medical and radiation oncologists.

During these detailed consultations, the family receives a thorough review of the pros and cons of treatments beyond the scope of the navigator's practice. They all have a much better understanding of why certain treatment options are and are not advised. This alleviates the initial concerns brought to the navigator's attention by R.M.'s daughter.

## Summary and Key Points

Patients and families faced with newly diagnosed prostate cancer are initially overwhelmed with the amount of information and the myriad treatment options available. Within the healthcare team, the nurse navigator can offer a unique role that addresses treatment decision making with patient perspective and understanding as the priorities. This optimizes patient satisfaction, quality of life, and care transitions.

- Patient education on treatment guidelines and facilitating shared decision making are tasks best served by the prostate cancer nurse navigator.
- Shared decision-making tools are readily available to help guide the navigator's counseling of patients and families facing prostate cancer.
- In addition to clinical indicators, quality of life and patient preferences should be included in any risk–benefit analysis in treatment decision making.

## Questions

### What is the primary goal of ADT for clinically localized, intermediate-risk prostate cancer?

The primary goal of ADT is to promote overall survival when given before, during, or after radiation therapy (e.g., neoadjuvant, concomitant, adjuvant ADT).

## What is an expected side effect of EBRT when used as primary therapy for prostate cancer?

An expected side effect of EBRT is fatigue during the final two weeks (Kazer & Harmon, 2011).

## References

Daugherty, P., Messier, N.G., dela Rama, F., Stern, H., Keen, S.J., & Blaseg, K.D. (2014). Cancer site–specific navigation. In K.D. Blaseg, P. Daugherty, & K.A. Gamblin (Eds.), *Oncology nurse navigation: Delivering patient-centered care across the continuum* (pp. 137–174). Pittsburgh, PA: Oncology Nursing Society.

Kazer, M.W., & Harmon, A.S. (2011). Radiation therapy: Toxicities and management. In C.H. Yarbro, D. Wujcik, & B.H. Gobel (Eds.), *Cancer nursing: Principles and practice* (7th ed., pp. 1609–1633). Burlington, MA: Jones & Bartlett Learning.

National Comprehensive Cancer Network. (2016). *NCCN Clinical Practice Guidelines in Oncology (NCCN Guidelines®): Prostate cancer* [v.3.2016]. Retrieved from http://www.nccn.org/professionals/physician_gls/pdf/prostate.pdf

Ottawa Hospital Research Institute. (2015). Ottawa personal decision guides. Retrieved from https://decisionaid.ohri.ca/decguide.html

Palo Alto Medical Foundation. (2010). *Chapter 4. Shared decision making process: Prioritizing goals for treatment and outcomes.* Retrieved from http://www.pamf.org/prostate/resources/binder.html

# Osteosarcoma and Mucositis in an Adolescent Patient

Paula Sanborn, RN, BSN, CPHON®

M.M. is a 16-year-old girl who comes to the clinic one week after receiving high-dose chemotherapy for osteosarcoma of the left proximal tibia. This is a scheduled visit to check laboratory values and perform an assessment. It is noted in the patient record that the physician on-call for the past weekend had received a call from M.M.'s grandmother stating that M.M. had not eaten in two days and was unable to take her medications by mouth due to mouth sores. The physician on-call instructed M.M. to come to the emergency department (ED) for evaluation, but she did not show.

During the initial intake interview, M.M. is unable to answer questions because of pain and swelling of her lips and oral mucosa. M.M.'s grandmother confirms that M.M. has consumed little food or liquid in three days and has been unable to take most of her medications due to the mouth pain. The grandmother states M.M. refused to come to the ED because it was the holiday weekend and she wanted to visit with family.

## What should the oncology nurse navigator (ONN) ask M.M. to adequately assess her oral mucosa and hydration status?

To further assess level of mucositis, M.M. is given a piece of paper and a pen to write down the answers to the ONN's questions, as it is too painful for her to talk. M.M. is asked the following:

- When did you first notice the mouth sores?
- Do you feel like the mouth sores are in the back of your throat?
- Has it been difficult to swallow?
- Does it hurt all the way down your throat?
- Are you having any difficulty breathing?
- Do you have an increase in oral secretions or any bleeding in your mouth or stools?
- Do you have any other symptoms, such as fever, chills, nausea, or vomiting (see Figure 14-1)?

## What should the ONN do next?

At this point, the ONN refers to the patient's medical record to verify the date of treatment, chemotherapy drugs received, and any medications M.M. was prescribed to take at home. The ONN asks the patient and her grandmother about the instructions they were given for taking medications to control mucositis. They also review the medical record for any comorbid conditions and a current medication list for any contributing factors. One week prior, M.M. had received week 32 (out of 40 weeks) of chemotherapy. She had been given high-dose methotrexate IV ($12 \text{ g/m}^2$) in week 31 and was readmitted three days later for ifosfamide $2.8 \text{ g/m}^2/$ day for five days in combination with etoposide $100 \text{ mg/m}^2/\text{day}$ for five days.

| Figure 14-1. Oral Mucositis Grading | | | | |
|---|---|---|---|---|
| 1 | 2 | 3 | 4 | 5 |
| Asymptomatic or mild symptoms; intervention not indicated | Moderate pain; not interfering with oral intake; modified diet indicated | Severe pain; interfering with oral intake | Life-threatening consequences; urgent intervention indicated | Death |

*Note.* From *Common Terminology Criteria for Adverse Events* [v.4.03], by National Cancer Institute Cancer Therapy Evaluation Program, 2010. Retrieved from http://evs.nci.nih.gov/ftp1/CTCAE/About/html.

It was noted at the time of discharge that M.M. had multiple 2 mm oral ulcerations with erythema (bilateral buccal mucosa). M.M. was instructed to take oxycodone 10 mg PO as needed every four hours for her mouth pain and inability to eat or take medications. She was told to use Weisman's Philadelphia Mouthwash (commonly referred to as "Magic Mouthwash"), a compounded mouthwash of diphenhydramine/aluminum-magnesium and hydroxide/lidocaine/water, at 10 ml per swish and spit every three hours for pain and prior to eating or taking oral medications. M.M. also was instructed to take fluconazole 200 mg PO once a day for 14 days until her white blood cell count recovered. The patient and her grandmother were reminded to call if M.M.'s mouth sores worsened or if her pain was not relieved by the regimen.

## What should the plan of care be?

The patient is further assessed with a physical examination and a measure of her vital signs. M.M. has a compromised airway. Pain control measures are initiated. The rest of her gastrointestinal tract is assessed for signs and symptoms of infection, such as nausea, vomiting, esophagitis, or bloody mucous stools.

M.M.'s physical assessment reveals bilateral oral lesions in the buccal mucosa; her palate and tongue are thick and coated in white patches. She has erythema of the gums, a throat tender to palpitation, and pain with swallowing. M.M. is pale with poor skin turgor and fatigue. She has an episode of epistaxis lasting 15 minutes during the examination. M.M. reports that her last urine output was the prior evening and it was dark golden yellow in color. She denies any diarrhea, but she has experienced an increase in thickened oral secretions. Vital signs include the following:

- Temperature—101°F (38°C)
- Pulse—149 beats per minute
- Respirations—26 breaths per minute
- Blood pressure—106/72 mm Hg
- Weight—down 6.8 lbs (3.1 kg) from discharge
- Pain scale rating—9.5/10 in mouth and throat

Because M.M. has not eaten in three days, is actively bleeding from her nose, is febrile, and is presenting with grade 3 mucositis, her port is accessed and laboratory tests are drawn, including blood cultures, complete blood count, type and screen, and chemistries (see Figure 14-2).

### Figure 14-2. Laboratory Results

- White blood cell count = 0.1 K/mm$^3$ (reference range 4.8–10.8)
- Hemoglobin = 6.5 g/dl (reference range 12–16)
- Platelets = 14 K/mm$^3$ (reference range 150–450)
- Absolute neutrophil count = 1 K/mm$^3$ (reference range 2.1–7.5)
- Sodium = 136 mmol/L (reference range 132–146)
- Potassium = 3.3 mmol/L (reference range 3.5–5.1)
- Chloride = 112 mmol/L (reference range 99–109)
- Carbon dioxide = 19 mmol/L (reference range 20–31)
- Calcium = 8.1 mg/dl (reference range 8.6–10.0)
- Magnesium = 1.6 mg/dl (reference range 1.5–1.5)
- Phosphorus = 2.9 mg/dl (reference range 2.5–4.5)
- Blood urea nitrogen = 26 mg/dl (reference range 9–23)
- Creatinine = 0.55 mg/dl (reference range 0.6–1.1)

*Note.* Reference ranges based on those in use at the time of this writing at Nationwide Children's Hospital, Columbus, OH.

After receiving laboratory results, the physician orders 1 liter of IV fluid to be administered over an hour and a morphine sulfate IV for pain. M.M. is admitted to the oncology unit for pain management, dehydration, and mucositis and to rule out sepsis (see Figure 14-3).

## What patient teaching is appropriate for this patient and her family?

During admission, M.M. admits she does not brush her teeth daily, use her mouth rinse, or take her pain medications regularly. Prior to discharge, the patient and her grandmother are instructed on daily oral care regimens and are provided with new soft toothbrushes, oral sponges, and desensitizing toothpaste. The patient and grandmother also are instructed on how to make sodium bicarbonate mouthwash (a mixture of ¼ teaspoon of salt, ¼ teaspoon of baking soda, and 4 ounces of water).

For a pain regimen, the ONN instructs M.M. to take oxycodone hydrochloride 20 minutes prior to eating or taking oral medications and using the prescribed mouthwash immediately prior to eating. The ONN also reviews the common signs and symptoms of dehydration, such as decreased urine output; dark urine; a dry, pasty mouth; and decreased skin turgor. The ONN instructs the patient and her grandmother to call if these symptoms occur.

---

### Figure 14-3. Treatment Plan

**Mucositis**
- Change all medications to IV.
  - Piperacillin/tazobactam IV
  - Fluconazole IV
  - Acyclovir IV (history of herpes simplex virus lesions)

**Thrombocytopenia**
- Transfuse platelets for < 20,000 or active bleeding.
- Obtain complete blood count (CBC) daily.

**Anemia**
- Administer packed red blood cell transfusion for hemoglobin < 8 g/dl.
- Obtain CBC daily.

**Dehydration**
- Provide maintenance IV fluids with potassium.
- Provide electrolyte infusions.
- Maintain regular diet; may transition to total parenteral nutrition, if indicated.
- Obtain daily chemistries, blood draw.

**Pain**
- Consult pain team.
  - Hydromorphone hydrochloride patient-controlled analgesia
  - Naloxone drip
  - IV acetaminophen PRN
  - Magic Mouthwash, as ordered
  - Sodium bicarbonate mouthwash, as scheduled

---

Oral care of the mouth includes the following:
- Brush teeth four times a day, including after meals and before bedtime with a soft toothbrush. Special instructions are given to patients who drink high-sugar sports drinks, requesting they brush after drinking these.
- Use only alcohol-free mouthwashes if desired.
- Examine the mouth daily for any signs of mucositis, looking at the entire mouth—lips, gums, tongue, sides of the tongue, under the tongue, cheeks, roof of the mouth, and around the teeth.
- Keep the mouth moist by eating Popsicles®, ice chips, slushies, smoothies, and cool fluids.
- Avoid spicy, bitter, salty, or acidic foods (Murphy, 2011) (see Figure 14-4).

**Figure 14-4. Food Considerations Regarding Mucositis**

| General Guidelines | Recommended | Not Recommended |
|---|---|---|
| • Small pieces of food<br>• Straws with liquids<br>• Nutritional supplements (e.g., Boost®, Scandishake®, Ensure®)<br>• Topical analgesics prior to eating<br>• Mouthwash (without alcohol) following meals<br>• Avoid hot foods. | • Tepid or cool liquids<br>• Puddings, Jell-O®<br>• Cottage cheese, soft cheeses<br>• Bananas, peaches, applesauce<br>• Milkshakes, smoothies<br>• Popsicles®, ice cubes, Italian water ice | • Spicy, salty, bitter foods<br>• Dry foods (e.g., crackers, toast, chips)<br>• Oranges, grapefruits, citrus fruits<br>• Chewing gum, candy |

## Summary and Key Points

M.M., a 16-year-old girl, experienced grade 3 mucositis. On arrival to the clinic, she was two weeks post high-dose methotrexate IV and one week post ifosfamide and etoposide for osteosarcoma of the left proximal tibia. Her mucositis was chemotherapy induced due to neutropenia, poor mouth care, and medication noncompliance. Laboratory findings indicated fluid and electrolyte imbalance, poor intake, and a history of acute kidney injury secondary to cisplatin and ifosfamide infusions, which were significant enough to require IV replacement. Physical presentation of a pain scale rating of 9.5/10 and the inability to open her mouth were significant factors, warranting hospital admission for pain control, IV fluids, and antibiotics. This hospitalization continued until M.M. reached adequate count recovery, was afebrile, and was able to take her nutrition and medications orally. Further treatment was delayed by one week. Doses were not modified because of her history of not being able to receive concurrent cisplatin due to hearing loss and removing doxorubicin from her treatment plan because of the risks of cardiotoxicity. The ONN took into account that M.M. is an adolescent and strived to maintain autonomy. M.M. was placed into the guardianship of her grandmother just prior to diagnosis, so reteaching of mouth care and medication adherence was vital. This education were completed at a time designated by the patient. A return visit was scheduled to demonstrate proper mouth care. Mouth care and medication adherence also was taught separately to her grandmother for continuity of care and to ensure of adherence to the plan of care.

- Chemotherapy agents inhibit the growth and maturation of oral mucosal cells and disrupt the primary mucosal barrier in the mouth and throat (Cripe & Yeager, 2015; Wohlschlaeger, 2004).
- These changes can occur as early as 2–3 days after the administration of chemotherapy and peak in severity 7–10 days later, typically showing resolution within two weeks (Cripe & Yeager, 2015; Wohlschlaeger, 2004).
- Chemotherapeutic agents that cause mucositis are listed in Table 14-1.
- Oral mucositis can cause impaired nutrition, infection leading to sepsis, and treatment delays (Baggott, Kelly, Fochtman, & Foley, 2002; Cripe & Yeager, 2015; Eilers & Million, 2011).

### Table 14-1. Chemotherapeutic Agents Causing Mucositis

| Drug Class | Agents |
|---|---|
| Alkylating agents | Busulfan<br>Cyclophosphamide<br>Ifosfamide<br>Melphalan<br>Procarbazine<br>Temozolomide<br>Thiotepa |
| Anthracyclines | Daunomycin<br>Doxorubicin<br>Idarubicin<br>Mitoxantrone |
| Antimetabolites | Cytarabine<br>5-Fluorouracil<br>Hydroxyurea<br>Mercaptopurine<br>Methotrexate<br>Thioguanine |
| Antineoplastic antibiotics | Bleomycin sulfate<br>Dactinomycin |
| Nitrosoureas | Carmustine<br>Lomustine |
| Plant alkaloids | Etoposide<br>Paclitaxel<br>Vinblastine<br>Vincristine |

Note. Based on information from Cripe & Yeager, 2015.

- Inadequate oral intake can lead to electrolyte abnormalities, such as sodium, potassium, calcium, magnesium, and phosphorus, especially in patients who have a history of electrolyte imbalance secondary to acute kidney injury related to high-dose cisplatin and ifosfamide infusions.
- Severe mucositis leading to an active infection also may lead to bone marrow suppression and decreased blood counts, such as white blood cells, hemoglobin, and platelets.
- Emerging data support the notion that adolescents and young adults (AYAs) should be treated as a subspecialty.
- AYAs are caught between the pediatric and the adult settings. They experience a different journey compared to their younger and older counterparts (Williams, 2013).
- AYAs are dealing with concepts such as autonomy and developing a set of values and relationships. This is a difficult time where control is lost. AYAs are forced to depend on family when they want to transition to independence (Williams, 2013).
- AYAs may make choices during their treatment that seem irresponsible. It is important to keep this in mind when having to reinstruct or reteach an already reviewed concept, as they are still cognitively maturing (Williams, 2013).
- Maintaining an open and developmentally appropriate communication style that avoids condescension will help foster compliance (Williams, 2013).

## Questions

### What concepts of growth and development should be considered when providing preventive measures for mucositis to an AYA patient?

AYA patients are dealing with developmental tasks (e.g., autonomy), but many times they are forced to depend on family when they desire to transition to independence (Williams, 2013).

### What oral care regimen is emphasized after receiving a chemotherapy agent that disrupts the mucosal barrier in the mouth and throat?

The routine that is emphasized includes brushing teeth four times a day (e.g., after meals, after drinking high-sugar drinks, at bedtime) and performing a thorough examination of the mouth. It is important to avoid spicy foods and keep the mouth moist (Murphy, 2011).

# References

Baggott, C.R., Kelly, K.P., Fochtman, D., & Foley, G.V. (2002). *Nursing care of children and adolescents with cancer.* Philadelphia, PA: Elsevier Saunders.

Cripe, T.P., & Yeager, N.D. (2015). *Malignant pediatric bone tumors—Treatment and management.* New York, NY: Springer.

Eilers, J., & Million, R. (2011). Clinical update: Prevention and management of oral mucositis in patients with cancer. *Seminars in Oncology Nursing, 27,* e1–e16. doi:10.1016/j.soncn.2011.08.001

Murphy, K. (Ed.). (2011). *The Children's Oncology Group family handbook for children with cancer.* Monrovia, CA: The Children's Oncology Group.

Williams, K.A. (2013). Adolescent and young adult oncology. *Clinical Journal of Oncology Nursing, 17,* 292–296. doi:10.1188/13.CJON.292-296

Wohlschlaeger, A. (2004). Prevention and treatment of mucositis: A guide for nurses. *Journal of Pediatric Oncology Nursing, 21,* 281–287. doi:10.1177/1043454204265840

# CASE 15
# Rhabdomyosarcoma in a Pediatric Patient

Paula Sanborn, RN, BSN, CPHON®

J.S. is a four-year-old developmentally delayed boy who comes to the clinic three days after receiving his second cycle of chemotherapy for rhabdomyosarcoma of the right masticator and pterygomaxillary space with parameningeal involvement. This is a scheduled visit to check laboratory values, receive his next dose of vincristine, and perform a nursing assessment. The visit also coincides with the fifth week of J.S.'s radiation treatments. During his intake assessment, J.S.'s mother reports he has been having loose stools for three days. She details giving him two or three doses of loperamide over the last three days without diarrhea resolution. J.S. also had a gastrostomy tube (g-tube) used for feedings and medication administration inserted prior to starting therapy. J.S.'s mother reports she has not been giving him extra feeds or hydration during his episodes of diarrhea and that he has been refusing anything orally. J.S. is having 6–8 liquid stools per day.

## What should the oncology nurse navigator (ONN) ask J.S. and his mother to adequately assess the loose stools?

To further assess the diarrhea, the ONN asks J.S.'s mother about J.S.'s usual number of stools per day, including stool consistency, color, odor, and the presence of blood or mucus. Clinicians use the number of stools over baseline to determine the severity of diarrhea (see Figure 15-1). The ONN also inquires if J.S. is having other

| Figure 15-1. Diarrhea Grading | | | | |
|---|---|---|---|---|
| 1 | 2 | 3 | 4 | 5 |
| Increase of < 4 stools per day over baseline; mild increase in ostomy output compared to baseline | Increase of 4–6 stools per day over baseline; moderate increase in ostomy output compared to baseline | Increase of ≥ 7 stools per day over baseline; incontinence, hospitalization indicated; severe increase in ostomy output compared to baseline, limiting self-care activities of daily living | Life-threatening consequences; urgent intervention indicated | Death |

Note. From *Common Terminology Criteria for Adverse Events* [v.4.03], by National Cancer Institute Cancer Therapy Evaluation Program, 2010. Retrieved from http://ctep.cancer.gov/protocolDevelopment/electronic_applications/ctc.htm.

symptoms, such as fever, chills, abdominal pain, bloating, nausea and vomiting, or decreased appetite or activity, or if anyone in the household has been ill.

## What should the ONN do next?

- Verify J.S.'s treatment schedule, including treatment dates and chemotherapy regimen.
- Perform a medication reconciliation to assess for any additional medications being taken at home.
- Evaluate J.S.'s activity level and sleep patterns.
- Ask about J.S.'s urinary output.
- Assess J.S.'s oral intake and nutrition status via his g-tube.
- Assess J.S.'s usual bowel pattern.
- Assess for mucositis and increased oral secretions caused by radiation therapy.
- Review previous instructions regarding treatment for diarrhea.

J.S.'s family is instructed to give him a dose of loperamide 2 mg (two teaspoons or one caplet) after his first loose bowel movement, followed by 1 mg (one teaspoonful or one-half caplet) every three hours. During the night, J.S. also can take 2 mg (two teaspoons or one caplet) every four hours, not exceeding 8 mg per day (Wagner et al., 2008). The family is instructed to call the clinic or the on-call physician if J.S. still has diarrhea after taking loperamide for 24 hours, has a fever, or is vomiting. The ONN emphasizes giving loperamide at the first sign of diarrhea and instructs J.S.'s mother to give doses as prescribed around the clock, including through the night and until J.S. does not have a stool movement for 12 hours.

If J.S. still has diarrhea after 24 hours of continuous treatment, the ONN instructs J.S.'s mother to call. His mother is reminded to stop all other stool softeners, such as Colace® and Senna®, and to use his g-tube to maintain hydration during diarrhea episodes (by giving Pedialyte® 3–4 ounces every 4–6 hours). J.S.'s mother also is given an educational tool for diarrhea (see Figure 15-2).

## What should be the plan of care?

J.S. undergoes a physical examination and has his vital signs checked. He is assessed for infectious diarrhea versus chemotherapy-induced diarrhea. The rest of J.S.'s gastrointestinal tract is assessed for signs and symptoms of infection, such as fever, chills, abdominal pain, cramping, lethargy, and abdominal tenderness. His oral mucosa is examined because of his concurrent radiation therapy.

J.S.'s physical assessment is remarkable for hyperactive bowel sounds and mild abdominal distention without tenderness. His skin turgor is poor. Oral mucosa is positive for erythema at the right buccal pouch and tender to touch on examination. J.S. has a small, loose, bloodless stool during the examination. It is odorless with no mucus present.

Vital signs are established and it is noted that J.S.'s weight is down 3.9 lbs (1.8 kg) from the previous week. J.S. describes a pain scale rating of 6 on the Wong-Baker FACES Pain Rating Scale (see Figure 15-3).

Because J.S. has been refusing oral intake, is lethargic, and presents with grade 3 diarrhea, an order is obtained for a complete blood count and chemistries drawn from his already accessed port, which is used daily for sedation with his radiation treatments. He also is monitored for fever, chills, and other signs of sepsis (see Figure 15-4).

After receiving laboratory results, the physician orders ondansetron 2 mg IV; hydrocodone-acetaminophen 2.5 mg–108 mg/5 ml oral solution, given 5 ml per g-tube; and g-tube bolus feed of Pedialyte 240 ml.

The physician does not order an IV fluid bolus because of a hemoglobin level of 8.9 g/dl and the potential of causing hyper-

---

**Figure 15-2. Nationwide Children's Hospital Diarrhea Education Tool**

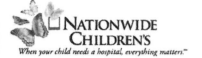

**Helping Hand**™

### Diarrhea

Diarrhea (loose, watery bowel movements) is a common problem of young children. Diarrhea may be caused by a serious illness, but usually it is only the result of a common viral infection.

The biggest danger of your child having diarrhea is that he can become dehydrated (dee-Hi-dray-ted). Dehydrated means that he gets very sick by losing too much fluid and getting "dried out." Dehydration can usually be prevented by increasing the amount of liquid a child drinks. We have examined your child and think that the diarrhea can be managed at home. You may need to give extra liquids more often, but in smaller amounts while your child is sick. Look below to see how to give him liquids.

### Liquids to Give

| Children younger than 1 year of age: | Children older than 1 year of age |
|---|---|
| • Pedialyte® or another balanced electrolyte solution, such as Infalyte®, Naturalyte®, Rehydralyte®, or Kao Lectrolyte® (powdered rehydration mix). These products are sold at most pharmacies without a prescription.<br>• Breast milk or formula | • Pedialyte® (any flavor)<br>• Ice pops<br>• Water<br>• Flavored gelatin cubes |

DO NOT give children of any age undiluted fruit juice or Kool-Aid® or soda.

### Amount of Liquid to Give
**Give the following amounts of the appropriate liquids based on your child's weight.**

| Child's Weight | Amount of Liquid to Give Every Hour |
|---|---|
| 7–10 pounds | 2 ounces (4 tablespoons) |
| 11–15 pounds | 2½ ounces (6 tablespoons) |
| 16–20 pounds | 3¼ ounces (½ of a large glass) |
| 21–40 pounds | 6½ ounces (one large glass) |
| 41–60 pounds | 10 ounces (1½ large glasses) |

*Note.* Figure courtesy of Nationwide Children's Hospital. Used with permission.

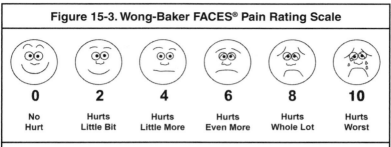

**Figure 15-3. Wong-Baker FACES® Pain Rating Scale**

| 0 | 2 | 4 | 6 | 8 | 10 |
|---|---|---|---|---|---|
| No Hurt | Hurts Little Bit | Hurts Little More | Hurts Even More | Hurts Whole Lot | Hurts Worst |

*Note.* Figure courtesy of Wong-Baker FACES® Foundation. Used with permission.

---

**Figure 15-4. Laboratory Results**

- White blood cell count = 1.4 K/mm$^3$ (reference range 4.8–10.8)
- Hemoglobin = 8.9 g/dl (reference range 12–16)
- Platelets = 207 K/mm$^3$ (reference range 150–450)
- Absolute neutrophil count = 560 K/mm$^3$ (reference range 2.1–7.5)
- Sodium = 139 mmol/L (reference range 132–146)
- Potassium = 3.8 mmol/L (reference range 3.5–5.1)
- Chloride = 111 mmol/L (reference range 99–109)
- Carbon dioxide = 20 mmol/L (reference range 20–31)
- Calcium = 9.5 mg/dl (reference range 8.6–10)
- Magnesium = 2.2 mg/dl (reference range 1.5–2.5)
- Phosphorus = 5.1 mg/dl (reference range 2.5–4.5)
- Blood urea nitrogen = 16 mg/dl (reference range 9–23)
- Creatinine = 0.39 mg/dl (reference range 0.6–1.1)
- Glucose = 84 mg/dl (reference range 70–139)

*Note.* Reference ranges based on those in use at the time of this writing at Nationwide Children's Hospital, Columbus, OH.

---

dilution of hemoglobin. J.S.'s family members are Jehovah's Witnesses and do not consent to blood transfusions. After a fluid bolus through his g-tube, an ondansetron dose, and pain medication, J.S. is more alert and active and has no further stools.

## What patient teaching is appropriate for J.S. and his family?

- If he is still experiencing diarrhea, wake J.S. at night every four hours for his dose of loperamide.
- Follow diarrhea management instructions (see Figure 15-5).

---

**Figure 15-5. Patient Instructions for Treating Irinotecan-Induced Diarrhea**

Your child is receiving irinotecan. This drug can cause severe diarrhea. Before your child's FIRST irinotecan treatment, please be sure to

1. BUY IMODIUM® A-D. Make sure you have this medication at home before your child's first Irinotecan treatment. Imodium A-D is also called LOPERAMIDE and comes in 2 mg caplets and in liquid form at a concentration of 0.2 mg/ml.
2. Throughout your child's treatment, the only way to recognize what diarrhea looks like is to compare bowel habits before and after treatment starts. Write down on the line below the number of bowel movements that your child has normally in a day or in a week and if the stool is normally hard or soft:

   _____ bowel movements per day OR
   _____ bowel movements per week
3. Stools usually appear

   _____ Hard _____ Loose _____ Formed _____ Soft _____ Watery
4. AFTER your child's irinotecan has started, be sure to note the following:
   Increase in number of stools? _____
   If so, how many? _____
   When did it start? _____
5. AFTER your child's irinotecan has started, be sure to START giving Imodium A-D at the FIRST SIGN of diarrhea. **DO NOT DELAY** starting Imodium A-D if you notice your child's stools to be more loose, soft, or watery than usual. Do not skip doses. Give Imodium A-D as instructed at the beginning of the first loose stool then every 3–4 hours as instructed, including waking your child during the night, and not exceeding the recommended daily dosing.
6. **STOP** giving Imodium A-D when your child **HAS NOT** had any bowel movements for 12 hours.
7. Call your doctor if your child still has diarrhea after taking Imodium A-D for 24 hours, or if there is fever or vomiting, or if you have any questions.
8. Your child's diarrhea can also get a little better with the following steps **IN ADDITION TO** taking Imodium A-D:
   • Drink plenty of water or Gatorade®.
   • Drink broth or clear soup to replace salt.
   • Stay away from milk, dairy products, alcohol, hot or cold beverages, coffee, tea, and drinks with caffeine.
9. Do not give your child medicines such as Miralax®, Mylanta®, Maalox®, Senokot®, or Colace®.
10. Have your child eat foods that are easy to tolerate, such as bananas, rice, applesauce, chicken (white meat), white toast, and canned fruits.

---

*Note.* Based on information from Sanborn, 2015.

- Look for signs and symptoms of dehydration, such as decreased urine output, less-wet diapers, dark urine, poor skin turgor, increased sleeping, and decreased activity.
- Continue with g-tube feedings with prescribed nutritional supplementation and allow J.S. to eat on demand during radiation treatments.
- Use a g-tube to maintain hydration during episodes of diarrhea, giving Pedialyte boluses three times a day.

J.S. is scheduled for a follow-up clinic appointment in three days. His mother is instructed to call if his diarrhea does not improve within 24 hours or if he develops a fever, pain, or increased lethargy. J.S.'s mother also is given a list of recommended foods that can help decrease diarrhea (Murphy, 2011) (see Figure 15-6).

## Summary and Key Points

J.S., a 4-year-old developmentally delayed boy, came to the clinic three days after receiving his second cycle of chemotherapy for rhabdomyosarcoma of the right masticator and pterygomaxillary space with parameningeal involvement. He had grade 3 diarrhea, which was most likely chemotherapy induced based on the pattern of occurrence and lack of contributing factors. Laboratory findings did not indicate fluid and electrolyte imbalance or severe dehydration.

| Figure 15-6. Foods and Beverages to Consume or Avoid During Episodes of Diarrhea | |
| --- | --- |
| **Recommended** | **Avoid** |
| • Water<br>• Sports drinks, such as Gatorade® or Powerade®<br>• Pedialyte® in liquid form or frozen pops<br>• Bananas<br>• Rice<br>• Applesauce<br>• Broth or chicken soup<br>• Chicken (preferably white meat)<br>• White toast<br>• Canned fruits | • Milk<br>• Dairy products<br>• Alcohol<br>• Hot or cold beverages<br>• Coffee<br>• Tea<br>• Soda<br>• Caffeinated beverages |

*Note.* From "Patient Navigation of the Pediatric Bone Tumor Patient Across the Continuum of Care" (p. 183), by P.M. Sanborn in T.P. Cripe and N.D. Yeager (Eds.), *Malignant Pediatric Bone Tumors—Treatment and Management, 2015,* New York, NY: Springer. Copyright 2015 by Springer. Adapted with permission.

Further treatment most likely will not be delayed unless his diarrhea progresses. Cefixime will be added to his treatment regimen five days prior to his next irinotecan cycle and will continue until day 21 (Wagner et al., 2008).

- Early-onset diarrhea typically occurs within four hours of irinotecan IV chemotherapy administration and is associated with cramping, flushing, and diaphoresis (extreme sweating).
  - Early-onset diarrhea is preventable or readily reversible with atropine administration and typically has not been dose-limiting (Wagner et al., 2008).
  - Late-onset diarrhea usually develops during the second week of therapy and can be dose-limiting, regardless of irinotecan chemotherapy administration schedule. One important factor is accumulation of the active metabolite SN-38 in the gut, causing direct cytotoxicity, local inflammation, and secretory diarrhea (Wagner et al., 2008).
- Chemotherapy-induced diarrhea can cause depletion of fluids and electrolytes, such as sodium, potassium, chloride, carbon dioxide, calcium, and magnesium; metabolic acidosis; malnutrition; dehydration; and hospitalization (Stein, Voigt, & Jordan, 2010).
- Chemotherapeutic agents that produce diarrhea are listed in Figure 15-7 (Baggott, Fochtman, Foley, & Kelly, 2011).
- The goal of diarrhea management is to restore normal bowel habits, maintain adequate nutrition, restore fluid and electrolyte balance, and maintain skin integrity (Baggott et al., 2011).
- The first step to diarrhea management is to monitor the amount and volume of stools by teaching the family to document how many stools the patient passes daily (Sanborn, 2015).
- Age-appropriate feeding is encouraged with oral rehydration solutions such as Pedialyte, which is given to replace excessive fluid loss in stool (Baggott et al., 2011).
- Topical skin barriers can be used in the pediatric population to maintain skin integrity (Baggott et al., 2011).
- Families are taught to recognize the signs and symptoms of dehydration and avoid hospitalization by being proactive in hydration techniques (Cripe & Yeager, 2015).
- As an ONN, it is important to respect cultural and religious beliefs and to become educated on varying patient backgrounds.
  - Jehovah's Witnesses believe that the Bible prohibits them from receiving blood products (e.g., red cells, white cells, platelets, plasma) and donating or storing their own blood for transfusion.

| Figure 15-7. Chemotherapy Agents Commonly Associated With Diarrhea |
| --- |

- Anthracyclines
  - Daunorubicin
  - Doxorubicin
- Antimetabolites
  - Cytosine arabinoside
  - 5-Fluorouracil
  - Methotrexate
  - Thioguanine
- Biologics
  - Interferon
  - Interleukin-2
- Cisplatin
- Cyclophosphamide
- Hydroxyurea
- Taxanes
  - Docetaxel
  - Paclitaxel
- Topoisomerase I inhibitors
  - Irinotecan
  - Topotecan
- Tyrosine kinase inhibitors
  - Gefitinib
  - Imatinib

*Note.* From "Managing Disease- and Treatment-Related Complications in Pediatric Oncology" (p. 536), by M.C. Hooke, D. Robinson, and A.M. Maloney in C. Baggott, D. Fochtman, G.V. Foley, and K.P. Kelly (Eds.), *Nursing Care of Children and Adolescents With Cancer and Blood Disorders* (4th ed.), 2011, Chicago, IL: Association of Pediatric Hematology/Oncology Nurses. Copyright 2011 by Association of Pediatric Hematology/Oncology Nurses. Reprinted with permission.

– Jehovah's Witnesses are taught that the use of fractions, such as albumin, immunoglobulins, and hemophiliac preparations, are not absolutely prohibited and are a matter of personal choice.

# Questions

### Early-onset diarrhea that occurs within four hours of administration of irinotecan is readily reversible with which drug?

It is reversible with atropine (Wagner et al., 2008).

## When did J.S.'s mother administer loperamide?

Late-onset diarrhea usually develops during the second week after irinotecan therapy and can be managed with home administration of loperamide. J.S.'s mother was instructed to start loperamide after the first loose stool and to continue dosing around the clock until her son does not have a bowel movement for 12 hours (Wagner et al., 2008).

# References

Baggott, C.R., Fochtman, D., Foley, G.V., & Kelly, K.P. (Eds.). (2011). *Nursing care of children and adolescents with cancer and blood disorders* (4th ed.). Chicago, IL: Association of Pediatric Hematology/Oncology Nurses.

Murphy, K. (2011). *The Children's Oncology Group family handbook for children with cancer.* Monrovia, CA: The Children's Oncology Group.

Sanborn, P.M. (2015). Patient navigation of the pediatric bone tumor patient across the continuum of care. In T.P. Cripe & N.D. Yeager (Eds.), *Malignant pediatric bone tumors—Treatment and management* (pp. 171–200). New York, NY: Springer.

Stein, A., Voigt, W., & Jordan, K. (2010). Review: Chemotherapy-induced diarrhea: Pathophysiology, frequency and guideline-based management. *Therapeutic Advances in Medical Oncology, 2*, 51–63. doi:10.1177/1758834009355164

Wagner, L.M., Crews, K.R., Stewart, C.F., Rodriguez-Galindo, C., McNall-Knapp, R.Y., Albritton, K., … Furman, W.L. (2008). Reducing irinotecan-associated diarrhea in children. *Pediatric Blood and Cancer, 50*, 201–207.

# Navigating a Patient With Multiple Disparities

Margaret Rummel, RN, MHA, OCN®, NE-BC

F.R. is a 53-year-old Spanish-speaking man who was diagnosed with squamous cell head and neck cancer (HNC) in 2011. He presents to the local emergency department with jaw pain and facial swelling, which he has had for several months. A computed tomography (CT) scan of the neck shows a mass in the left tonsillar area and soft palate. Because of the complexity of his disease, F.R. is referred to an academic medical center for further evaluation.

He meets with an ear, nose, and throat surgeon, who does a thorough medical history and physical examination. Results are unremarkable. F.R. has had no previous surgeries or comorbidities and is not on any routine medications. Preoperative laboratory values are all normal.

F.R. has an endoscopy and biopsy under local anesthesia. The biopsy confirms squamous cell HNC that is human papillomavirus (HPV) positive. F.R. is diagnosed with stage T4 N2 M0 squamous cell HNC because of the bony invasion of his jaw. The disease is extensive. Although the disease is resectable, the surgeon feels that a significant risk exists of a permanent swallowing deficit and disfigurement. After discussing the findings, F.R. is referred to the multidisciplinary oncology team. This team approach is very important to the successful treating of patients with HNC and maintaining good patient quality of life.

## What should the oncology nurse navigator (ONN) know about HNC?

HNC can occur in any part of the pharynx (a tube about five inches long, extending from the back of the nose to the area where the esophagus and the trachea both begin). The pharynx and surrounding structures are divided into several areas, including the oral cavity, nasopharynx, oropharynx, hypopharynx, larynx, sinuses, ear, and neck. HNC can occur in any of these areas (Cancer.Net, n.d.; Vachani, 2015).

F.R. is referred to the oncology clinic, where he meets with the medical and radiation oncologists and the ONN. It is recommended that he receive seven weeks of induction chemotherapy with carboplatin, paclitaxel, and cetuximab. This is followed by concurrent chemoradiation with cisplatin. Chemotherapy commonly is given in conjunction with radiation therapy. Chemotherapy treats the cancer cells and makes them more sensitive to the radiation. The induction chemotherapy shrinks the tumor prior to administration of other treatments.

A Spanish interpreter is present for all consults, as F.R.'s language barrier is the most significant obstacle he faces in understanding his disease and treatment course (Blaseg, Daugherty, & Gamblin, 2014; National Comprehensive Cancer Network® [NCCN®], 2016).

## What questions should the ONN ask to assess the patient's knowledge and understanding of the plan of care and treatment?

The ONN asks F.R. about his social situation and support system. On assessment, the ONN discovers F.R. lives alone and has very few friends and family. His closest relative is his cousin, who has his medical and legal power of attorney. On a lifestyle assessment, F.R. details that he smokes two packs of cigarettes and drinks a 12-pack of beer daily. The ONN encourages F.R. to go to smoking cessation classes and to stop drinking. F.R. declines and states that he is not interested in quitting at this time. Both behaviors are risk factors in the development of HNC. F.R. tells the ONN that these habits are "how he copes with life."

F.R. speaks and reads minimal English. The ONN determines that a medical interpreter will be present for all visits and that all written educational material will be in Spanish. F.R. does not drive and believes that getting back and forth to treatment will be a problem. Public transportation is available, but the ONN states that F.R.

will need a backup plan. F.R. relays that his cousin or a neighbor can occasionally drive him to treatment.

F.R.'s income is limited and he does not work. He lost his machinist job when the company went out of business. F.R. is underinsured and has no prescription coverage. He also states that he has a fear of doctors and hospitals, which is why he did not address his jaw pain earlier. In his culture, F.R. believes that it is not "manly" to complain about pain or to take any medications for pain. He says that he was "always told to be strong." F.R. has lost weight because of his inability to eat due to pain.

The ONN meets with F.R.'s cousin to review all instructions. To assist in his treatment, the ONN refers F.R. to the following resources:

- A social work consult to assist with social and logistical issues (e.g., transportation). F.R. is assigned a social work intern who speaks Spanish and is able to communicate with him on an ongoing basis. The intern provides support and counseling as needed.
- A nutrition consult to follow up on F.R.'s weight loss and provide education on his caloric needs during treatment. A local meal program is requested to provide F.R. with nutritious meals during treatment.
- An interpreter to be present for all visits
- A financial counselor to assist with F.R.'s lack of adequate insurance and prescription plan
- A smoking cessation clinic, which F.R. is not interested in attending
- A counselor for ongoing support and coping with body image changes

## What main teaching points should the ONN review with F.R. regarding his treatment plan?

The ONN reviews the side effects of the induction chemotherapy regimen, including rashes related to cetuximab, fever, malaise, peripheral neuropathy, hair loss, nausea and vomiting, and bone marrow depression. F.R. is instructed on when and how to take his medications for nausea and pain. He also is told to take an over-the-counter laxative if he has not had a bowel movement for two days. F.R. is prescribed a stool softener and is instructed to take two tablets on a daily basis. Instructions also are provided on skin care, as F.R. is receiving cetuximab, which can cause a rash (Vachani, 2015).

The ONN reviews all of these instructions with F.R.'s cousin so that she can help manage his care. F.R. is provided educational material written in Spanish on his drug regimen and side effects and is given instructions on when and how to contact his medical team. He agrees to call his cousin for problems and concerns. She will call his medical team, as she speaks both English and Spanish.

The ONN explains what to expect at F.R.'s weekly visits for chemotherapy. Even though radiation will not start for several weeks, the ONN initiates patient education regarding radiation therapy, as F.R. needs extensive teaching and constant reteaching regarding treatment.

While receiving induction chemotherapy, F.R. is set up with the following providers:

- Dentist—F.R. will receive an oral assessment, as radiation therapy can cause tooth decay. Damaged teeth may need to be removed prior to treatment. F.R. does not have dental coverage, so he is scheduled to see the county health clinic for his dental services and extractions. Because of his radiation treatments, he is given a prescription for sodium fluoride to be used daily.
- Speech pathologist—F.R. will undergo a preradiation speech and swallowing evaluation and will be provided with swallowing exercises that can be done during treatment.
- Gastroenterologist—If he is unable to maintain adequate nutrition during treatment, F.R. will be evaluated for a possible percutaneous endoscopic gastrostomy (PEG) tube.
- Audiologist—Prior to his cisplatin therapy, F.R. will receive a hearing test, as this agent can cause hearing problems. A baseline examination is needed to determine cisplatin dosing.

F.R. receives his loading dose of cetuximab. He returns for his second week of therapy. Based on a discussion with the ONN, F.R. clearly lacks understanding of the plan of care. His chemotherapy is held until the team can ensure his understanding.

Another educational session is scheduled. The team asks to have his cousin present for this meeting. His cousin comes for the session and treatment is resumed, as the team feels that F.R. better understands the plan of care.

Treatment is again held during the sixth week because of leukopenia. The ONN meets with F.R. every week to assess any additional barriers to care and his compliance with the treatment plan. The

ONN also provides support as F.R. undergoes treatment. F.R. is scheduled for his simulation and mask fitting prior to initiating external beam radiation. He is instructed on his treatment schedule, which is reviewed by the interpreter and social work intern. Side effects are discussed. F.R. is provided with an educational sheet on side effect management and instructions on when to call his team. Examples of side effect instructions can be found on OncoLink's website (www .oncolink.org/cancer-treatment/radiation/side-effects).

## What is the ONN's role once treatment is completed?

Once F.R. completes his chemotherapy and radiation treatments, he works with the ONN on developing a follow-up schedule; however, F.R. only shows for a few appointments. The ONN reaches out to F.R. and his cousin, but they do not return the calls.

## How can the ONN help F.R. when his disease recurs?

Two years later, F.R. calls his ONN with "horrible" pain and asks for assistance in getting an appointment. He reports that he has been taking escalating doses of pain narcotics, which he had been getting from various providers in his neighborhood. A magnetic resonance imaging (MRI) of the neck is done. It is concerning for disease recurrence with perineural spread.

After much discussion, F.R. agrees to have a left hemimandibulectomy with free flap reconstruction and a neck dissection. He has a tracheostomy and PEG tube placed during surgery. The pathology report is consistent with recurrent squamous cell HNC. The surgical margins are negative and no evidence of lymph node involvement is found. His postoperative course is uneventful. He is discharged to a rehabilitation facility close to home for additional recovery.

The ONN works closely with the rehabilitation facility to ensure that F.R. comes for his scheduled follow-up visits and testing. F.R. is referred to the palliative care team for help in managing his pain. Moving forward, it is important that only one provider is responsible for managing F.R.'s pain medications. This prevents him from receiving medications from multiple providers. F.R. also agrees to attend a smoking cessation program scheduled by his ONN.

F.R. is readmitted to the hospital twice after surgery for fluid accumulation at his wound site. He undergoes ultrasound-guided drainage of the wound twice before it heals. Cytology is negative. F.R. continues to recover from his surgery and is compliant with his follow-up care.

After his wound heals, the ONN schedules F.R. for lymphedema therapy to help with range of motion and postoperative edema. His trach and PEG tube are removed. He continues his regular follow-up with his providers and has no evidence of disease. The ONN periodically checks with F.R. and sees him at follow-up appointments. F.R.'s nutrition status remains stable, although he has stated that he has lost his taste for many foods. The oncology dietitian periodically checks in regarding his nutrition. F.R. is edentulous because of his altered anatomy, which limits his eating ability. The ONN provides assistance in getting dentures.

## Summary and Key Points

F.R., a 53-year-old Spanish-speaking man, was diagnosed with stage T4 N2 M0 squamous cell HNC. He underwent several courses of treatment, including surgery, chemotherapy, and radiation therapy. He had many barriers and obstacles to care, including transportation issues, social issues, language barriers, lack of understanding of the plan of care, and financial concerns. The ONN played a significant role in achieving positive outcomes and was able to implement a plan to assist the patient throughout the course of his disease.

The ONN also was able to think "outside the box" to help F.R. through his cancer journey. F.R. was connected with many helpful resources to achieve a successful outcome and provide support to his family.

- External beam radiation is the most commonly used form of radiation for HNC. Radiation not only targets the cancer, but it also affects nearby healthy cells, leading to side effects (e.g., sore mouth/throat [mucositis], dermatitis and painful swallowing, dry mouth or nose).
- Proton therapy is another type of radiation therapy used to treat HNC. This treatment limits side effects to healthy tissue because of the way the proton beam is delivered to the cancer. Not all patients are eligible for proton therapy, nor is it always the best treatment plan.

- HNCs account for approximately 3% of all cancers in the United States. These cancers are nearly twice as common in men as they are in women. They are diagnosed more often in people over the age of 50 (American Cancer Society, 2015).
- Alcohol and tobacco use, including smokeless tobacco (i.e., "chewing tobacco" or "snuff"), are the two most important risk factors for HNCs. People who use both tobacco and alcohol are at a greater risk for developing these cancers than people who use tobacco or alcohol alone (Carr, 2016).
- Infection with cancer-causing types of HPV, especially HPV-16, is a risk factor for some types of HNCs, particularly oropharyngeal cancers that involve the tonsils or the base of the tongue. HPV-positive cancers have a better outcome than HPV-negative cancers (Vachani, 2015).
- Early-stage HNCs (I and II) are treated with surgery with or without radiation (NCCN, 2016).
- Late-stage HNCs (III and IV) require treatment with multimodality therapies, including surgery, chemotherapy, and radiation (NCCN, 2016).
- Diagnosis is made by imaging, specifically a CT scan or MRI and positron-emission tomography scans. This is followed by endoscopy and biopsy of the affected area (NCCN, 2016).
- Pathology determines the type of HNC present and provides guidelines for treatment.

## Questions

### What risk factors placed F.R. at high risk for squamous cell HNC?

F.R. was a heavy smoker and alcohol user, which are two lifestyle behaviors that place patients at high risk for developing squamous cell HNC. People who use both tobacco and alcohol are at greater risk of developing these cancers than those who use either tobacco or alcohol (Vachani, 2015).

### What was the most significant barrier to care for F.R., and how was it overcome?

F.R.'s language barrier was the most significant obstacle to obtaining care. According to Freeman and Rodriguez (2011), communication is one of the top five barriers that patients encounter when receiving care and attempting to navigate the healthcare system. The ONN assigned a medical interpreter for all appointments to ensure communication.

## References

American Cancer Society. (2015). Oral cavity and oropharyngeal cancer. Retrieved from http://www.cancer.org/cancer/oralcavityandoropharyngealcancer

Blaseg, K.D. (2014). Getting started as a nurse navigator. In K.D. Blaseg, P. Daugherty, & K.A. Gamblin (Eds.), *Oncology nurse navigation: Delivering patient-centered care across the continuum* (pp. 15–42). Pittsburgh, PA: Oncology Nursing Society.

Cancer.Net. (n.d.). Head and neck cancer. Retrieved from http://www.cancer.net/cancer-types/head-and-neck-cancer

Carr, E. (2016). Head and neck cancers. In J.K. Itano (Ed.), *Core curriculum for oncology nursing* (5th ed., pp. 139–151). St. Louis, MO: Elsevier.

Freeman, H.P., & Rodriguez, R.L. (2011). History and principles of patient navigation. *Cancer, 117*(Suppl. 15), 3537–3540. doi:10.1002/cncr.26262

National Comprehensive Cancer Network. (2016). *NCCN Clinical Practice Guidelines in Oncology (NCCN Guidelines®): Head and neck cancers* [v.1.2016]. Retrieved from https://www.nccn.org/professionals/physician_gls/pdf/head-and-neck.pdf

Vachani, C. (2015). All about head and neck cancers. Retrieved from http://www.oncolink.org/types/article.cfm?c=243&aid=256&id=9545

# Overcoming the Financial and Emotional Barriers of Patients

Venteria L. Knight, RN, MPH

T.S. is a 38-year-old African American woman with no children. She is employed with a property management company, is single, and lives with her mother. T.S. has decent health insurance coverage despite a low income. She has no family history of cancer but decides to speak with her doctor to schedule a baseline screening mammogram.

T.S. worries about her results and the "what ifs" of possibly having cancer. It is one thing to take a day off work to attend appointments, but it is another for her to miss multiple days of work for a treatment that she cannot afford, especially when a day off can mean an unpaid household bill. Following a series of callbacks and attempts to fit appointments into her work schedule, a biopsy reveals a diagnosis of stage IIA cancer in her left breast. T.S. is referred to a surgeon.

## How can a navigator assist with the financial burden associated with a cancer diagnosis?

The cost of medical treatments is one of the most common concerns that patients and families face with a cancer diagnosis. This potentially leads to noncompliance with care and higher costs in the long run (Cancer.Net, 2015).

As part of facility protocol, T.S. is put in contact with a nurse navigator. During the initial conversation with the navigator, T.S. mentions that the medical bills leading up to her diagnosis have piled up and that she is having trouble with out-of-pocket expenses and co-pays. She is referred to a disparities nurse navigator for further financial assessment and discussion of resources.

T.S. has not had a consultation with the surgeon to discuss her treatment plan because of a high specialist co-pay for the visit. She normally is paid on the 1st and 15th of every month. Her last paycheck was used to cover household expenses and other medical bills. She plans to schedule an appointment after her next payday in two to three weeks. At this point, T.S. has not discussed her financial concerns with anyone other than her navigator.

T.S. is encouraged by the disparities navigator to contact her surgeon's office, explain the situation, and inquire about payment arrangements. The disparities navigator details the hospital's financial assistance program. T.S. also is referred to a local American Cancer Society (ACS) navigator for non–hospital-based resources.

T.S. receives 70% approval for financial assistance at the hospital. She has a lumpectomy scheduled in two months. T.S. declines neoadjuvant chemotherapy because of potential side effects and financial concerns. The financial assistance also finds T.S. genetic counseling and testing at a discounted price.

According to the U.S. Census Bureau, expenditures for cancer care could reach $158 billion by 2020. That is up from the estimated rate of $124 billion in 2010 (National Cancer Institute [NCI], 2011) (see Figure 17-1).

## How can navigation assist with fertility issues?

Some cancer treatments can affect a woman's ability to reproduce (ACS, 2013). T.S. has a desire to have children one day and is very interested in fertility. She contacts the disparities navigator about the possibility of financial assistance covering egg preservation and fertility treatments. Unfortunately, no financial assistance is available. The navigator is able to find some treatment centers that offer discounts and payment plans but nothing that T.S. can afford.

Although T.S. cannot find an option that is affordable, she at least is able to have the discussion with her navigator. If a physician does not bring up preservation of fertility, patients with cancer often may not feel comfortable discussing available options with their doctors. Patients may worry that the provider may not think fertility issues are important and that their physicians should be more focused on treatment and care (ACS, 2013).

It is imperative that patients feel comfortable talking to their healthcare team about any concerns. Early patient contact with nav-

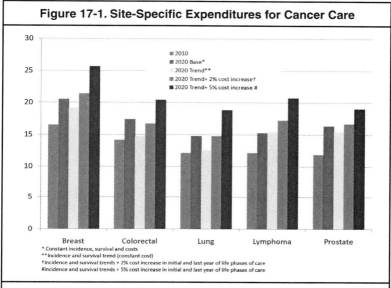

**Figure 17-1. Site-Specific Expenditures for Cancer Care**

\* Constant incidence, survival and costs
\*\*Incidence and survival trend (constant cost)
†Incidence and survival trends + 2% cost increase in initial and last year of life phases of care
#Incidence and survival trends + 5% cost increase in initial and last year of life phases of care

*Note.* From "Cancer Care Costs Predicted to Reach at Least $158 Billion in 2020," by National Cancer Institute, 2011. Retrieved from http://www.cancer.gov/news-events/press-releases/2011/CostCancer2020.

igation is crucial. The relationships that navigators build with their patients can encourage them to be more open and share more. The American Society of Clinical Oncology recommends that fertility options are discussed before therapy as part of the consent and education process for patients in their reproductive years (Lee et al., 2006). Some fertility and cancer resources include the following:

• American Cancer Society—www.cancer.org/index
• Livestrong—www.livestrong.org/we-can-help/fertility-services/fertility-hcps
• Reprotech—www.reprotech.com/fertility-preservation.html

## How can the navigator assist the caregiver?

While still in treatment, T.S. asks for some resources for her mother, who is uninsured and needs to have a mammogram and colonoscopy. T.S. is connected with a financial access surgery program and a free mammography program.

In the meantime, T.S. prepares for her own lumpectomy. She reports that she has been sleeping on a couch or air mattress and requests assistance with getting a bed. T.S. is concerned she will have a greater chance to contract an infection or develop lymphedema if she is not able to sleep in a proper bed. Her request is unusual for the disparities navigator, who asks the ACS navigator to help research options for the patient. In the end, the navigators are able to find a bed through help from a local church.

In January of the following year, the disparities navigator speaks to T.S. after not hearing from her for a while. T.S. has missed a scheduled appointment because her mother had to be rushed to the emergency department (ED).

A week later, T.S.'s uninsured mother is referred to the disparities navigator for financial assistance. Just seven months after T.S.'s diagnosis of breast cancer, her mother is diagnosed with metastatic high-grade serous carcinoma of the ovaries. She is a morbidly obese 55-year-old woman who came to the ED with shortness of breath, rashes on her face and chest, and anxiety. She has no past medical history other than gastroesophageal reflux disease. She is admitted to the hospital and remains for several weeks.

In the midst of T.S.'s cancer treatment, she has to start caring for her mother. Their family situation becomes worse. They lose their car and are evicted from their home. Their plans to move back to the West Coast with family fall through.

T.S. and her mother start chemotherapy. Transportation was previously arranged by the hospital through a program with a local taxi company. At that time, they lived 15 miles from the hospital. After they were evicted from their home, the mother and daughter moved in with friends nearly 40 miles away. Their new living arrangements make transportation an even bigger obstacle. Navigators try assisting T.S.'s mother with information to apply for disability payments, but because she owns willed property in a nearby rural town, she is not eligible. Navigation continues to help with transportation and wishes to get more supportive services to T.S. and her mother; however, they both refuse additional help.

## Summary and Key Points

In this case study, navigation addressed several disparities, including income, disability, and geographic location. Financial advocacy can be an integral part of any cancer program or care team and can save lives. This was demonstrated in Dr. Harold Freeman's program, where five-year survival was significantly increased in Harlem through promotion of cancer screening and assistance with financial support for treatment (Seagraves, 2007). One might think the burden of finances during cancer treatment should be the least of one's worries after a cancer diagnosis; however, patients with cancer may fear costs more than the cancer itself (Association of Community Cancer Centers, 2015).

Navigators who work in this area can help with transportation, medication co-pays, assistance with applying for hospital-based and drug company–based programs, and information on community resources. Financial navigators can be nurses, social workers, other healthcare professionals, or lay people. This is a situation where the professional, the patient, and caregivers can work together for the best interests of all.

Merriam-Webster defines the word *caregiver* as "a person who gives help and protection to someone (such as a child, an old person, or someone who is sick)" ("Caregiver", n.d.). Caregivers are commonly thought of as healthcare professionals; however, lay people, such as friends or family of the patient, are an essential part of the healthcare team. Those closest to the patient can effectively serve as caregivers by providing transportation, offering financial and psychological support, coordinating care, and providing cultural and language barrier assistance. More than 1.6 million new patients are expected to be diagnosed with cancer in the United States in 2016 (NCI, 2016). Many of them may require caregivers at some point. Taking care of someone who is ill can be an overwhelming task filled with worry, exhaustion, and anxiety. These symptoms double when the caregivers themselves are sick. Left with no support, these patients must rely on their cancer care team.

- When considering unusual requests (e.g., finding a bed), navigators sometimes look to the Internet for solutions. An example would be a navigator searching for items requested by a patient on Craigslist, eBay, or similar sites.
- Online communities are sometimes willing to donate items for a good cause.
- Navigation professionals and patients should never offer to meet anyone that they contact online in private. Always use a secure, public place to meet, such as a police station or fire department.

Navigators and patients should have a cell phone handy and tell someone else where they are going.

## Questions

### What steps should a patient or caregiver take to address the burden of financial concerns?

The first step is to voice concern early on. Proactive intervention can lessen emotional and financial burdens and allow for timely access to care (Seagraves, 2007). Community and national programs also are available; however, a waiting list may exist or applications may take a few weeks for approval. Many hospitals and medical practices have financial assistance programs that go unshared unless patients inquire about them. The healthcare team, including physicians, navigators, and social workers, is part of a trust circle. In this relationship, patients and caregivers should feel free to share concerns and ask questions without fear of judgment or retaliation. Caregivers often will take on additional burdens and not express their needs (Girgis, Lambert, Johnson, Waller, & Currow, 2013). There is no shame in asking for help. Power is found from being one's own advocate or advocating for a loved one.

### What are important considerations for caregivers of patients with cancer?

Caregiver stress and fatigue are among the highest reported effects of caring for patients with cancer (Bevans & Sternberg, 2012). Navigators can serve an important role in sharing information on how patients can take care of themselves. Including caregivers in this process is vital.

### Besides navigation, what other resources exist for caregivers?

Some institutions offer caregiver support groups or affiliations with other support organizations, such as Gilda's Club or the Cancer Support Community. Faith-based organizations are another great resource. Patients often can contact health or community ministries offering various types of aid. For patients who are tech savvy, CaringBridge (www.caringbridge.org) is a website that allows participants to connect and share status updates.

# References

American Cancer Society. (2013). Talking to your cancer team about fertility before your treatment. Retrieved from http://www.cancer.org/treatment/ treatmentsandsideeffects/physicalsideeffects/sexualsideeffectsinwomen/ fertilityandwomenwithcancer/fertility-and-women-with-cancer-talking-about -fertility

Association of Community Cancer Programs. (2015). Financial advocacy network case-based workshops. Retrieved from http://accc-cancer.org/resources/Financial Advocacy-Meetings.asp

Bevans, M.F., & Sternberg, E.M. (2012). Caregiving burden, stress, and health effects among family caregivers of adult cancer patients. *JAMA, 307,* 398–403. doi:10.1001/jama.2012.29

Cancer.Net. (2015). Introduction to the costs of cancer care. Retrieved from http:// www.cancer.net/navigating-cancer-care/financial-considerations/introduction -costs-cancer-care

Caregiver. (n.d.). In *Merriam-Webster's online dictionary.* Retrieved from http://www .merriam-webster.com/dictionary/caregiver

Girgis, A., Lambert, S., Johnson, C., Waller, A., & Currow, D. (2013). Physical, psychosocial, relationship, and economic burden of caring for people with cancer: A review. *Journal of Oncology Practice, 9,* 197–202. doi:10.1200/JOP.2012.000690

Lee, S., Schover, L.R., Partridge, A.H., Patrizio, P., Wallace, W.H., Hagerty, K., ... Oktay, K. (2006). American Society of Clinical Oncology recommendations on fertility preservation in cancer patients. *Journal of Clinical Oncology, 24,* 2917–2931. doi:10.1200/JCO.2006.06.5888

National Cancer Institute. (2011). Cancer care costs projected to reach at least $158 billion in 2020. Retrieved from http://www.cancer.gov/news-events/press -releases/2011/CostCancer2020

National Cancer Institute. (2016). Cancer statistics. Retrieved from http://www .cancer.gov/about-cancer/understanding/statistics

Seagraves, K. (2007). Unraveling the cancer-poverty connection. Retrieved from http://povertynewsblog.blogspot.com/2007/03/unraveling-cancer-poverty -connection.html

# CASE 18
# Transitioning to Palliative Care

Betty Ferrell, PhD, RN, FAAN, FPCN, and Tami Borneman, MSN, CNS, FPCN

J.S. is a 38-year-old married mother of two young children, ages 5 and 8. After seeking several additional opinions about diagnosis and treatment for stage IV non-small cell lung cancer, she decides to be treated at a comprehensive cancer center and is scheduled for her second chemotherapy treatment. J.S.'s family cancer history includes breast, lung, colon, prostate, cervical, brain, and melanoma. She and her husband want to do everything possible to extend her life. They are not open to a goals-of-care discussion or any discussion about end of life. They insist that their only focus is on treatment. J.S.'s main symptom complaint is pain, which she rates at 7/10. She also does not like the out-of-control feeling of pain medications. She has fatigue at 7/10, has a decreased appetite and a 20-pound weight loss, and is unable to perform most of her activities of daily living.

After J.S.'s third clinic visit and second chemotherapy treatment, the palliative care team is asked to be involved in J.S.'s care; however, before she is seen by this team, J.S. is hospitalized for back pain. During this hospitalization, members of the palliative care team, including a pain specialist, a social worker, and a chaplain, meet with J.S. and her husband to help navigate a plan of care and sort out treatment goals. Her pain is brought under control and she is discharged the next day.

## Why is it important to initially involve the palliative care team in care navigation?

Involving the palliative care team early in J.S.'s treatment provides the best approach to whole patient care and navigation. The palliative care team works concurrently with the physician and nurse to address J.S.'s many needs. With a focus on addressing pain and symptom management, providing psychosocial support, and facilitating informed decisions, palliative care can improve quality of life and reduce unneeded medical services (Bakitas et al., 2009; Temel et al., 2010). Metastatic lung cancer carries a high symptom burden and poor quality of life. Providing early palliative care has been shown to improve survival when compared to standard care alone (Temel et al., 2010).

J.S. is sad and very tearful. Both she and her husband resist talking about their children. They want to protect them at all costs. To this point, they have not informed them of the severity of J.S.'s illness. They maintain a positive outlook at home and decline offers for help. J.S. and her husband have supportive friends but not many who live close to them. J.S. has a strained relationship with her mother and sisters. She also tends to isolate herself from her kids and often is unable to care for them. Consequently, her mother has come to help with the children. J.S. relies on her husband for both emotional and physical support.

## How might a family conference educate about the guidance role of the palliative care team?

The goal of having a family conference at this time serves several purposes. First, it is important to clarify what palliative care is and what it is not, as many patients confuse palliative care with hospice care. The team explains that providing palliative care concurrently with treatment is providing standard care (Dahlin, 2013). The care team can aggressively manage J.S.'s pain and any other possible symptoms.

In addition, the family conference empowers J.S. and her husband to share their feelings and frustrations and to clarify previously unclear information (Fineberg & Bauer, 2011). In general, the family conference is intended to provide an opportunity for shared understanding.

The social worker begins the conversation with J.S. and her husband about their children. This is a very delicate issue, as the couple does not want their children to know the extent of their mother's illness. In these situations, a child life specialist can be very helpful. These specialists are trained pediatric healthcare professionals who work with children and families in hospitals and other settings, helping them to cope with the challenges of hospitalization, illness, and other life events (Child Life Council, n.d.). In wanting what is best for the children, the social worker also can plant the seed for an advance directive. The team can support patients' spouses by providing resources.

## When should the team chaplain be involved in the care trajectory?

Unless specifically refused, the team chaplain and other team members should be involved from the beginning of care. When chaplains are introduced as part of the team, it helps to remove the stigma sometimes associated with offering clergy services.

Even though J.S. and her husband are not active in their faith, they both believe in prayer. Despite not being an active churchgoer, J.S. welcomes the chaplain. She simultaneously is angry with God and believes his love to be unconditional. She states, "I cannot stand to see the pain in my children's eyes."

J.S. shares her anger at God. She debates what to tell her children. J.S. is afraid of not seeing them grow up. She expresses guilt about leaving her husband alone. J.S. is clearly experiencing spiritual distress.

The chaplain states that the team will not give up on or abandon her or her family. The chaplain schedules another visit with J.S. and provides her with his business card. The importance of assessing spirituality has come to the forefront of research over the past decade. The National Consensus Project for Quality Palliative Care (Dahlin, 2013) identified eight domains of palliative care, with the fifth domain addressing spiritual, religious, and existential aspects of care. Held in 2009, the National Consensus Conference provided a definition for spirituality: "Spirituality is the aspect of humanity that refers to the way individuals seek and express meaning and purpose, and the way they experience their connectedness to the moment, to self, to others, to nature and to the significant or sacred" (Puchalski & Ferrell, 2010, p. 25).

## How does the primary care role transition to the palliative care team?

Initially, J.S.'s treatments work. She enjoys about four months of fairly good quality of life.

After her initial treatments are no longer effective, other treatment regimens are attempted but are not successful. J.S. begins having seizures from brain metastases and chooses to have surgery for an Ommaya shunt placement. Her husband rarely leaves her side and is exhausted. J.S.'s mother is still taking care of the children.

The medical oncologist and nurse work closely with the palliative care team throughout J.S.'s treatment. Several unsuccessful attempts are made by the oncologist, nurse, and social worker to discuss an advance directive. While J.S. and her husband are open to palliative care team visits, they are not always willing to accept their recommendations. J.S. refuses pain medications at a dosage that alleviates her pain, as it makes her too drowsy. Whatever the oncologist and nurse engage in with J.S. and her husband, the palliative care team reinforces and vice versa. Everyone on the whole team is on the same page.

Most patients have a very hard time accepting that treatment is no longer working and all options have been exhausted. It is at this juncture of J.S.'s disease progression that the palliative care team is asked to take over J.S.'s care completely. Because J.S. and her husband will not relent on the idea of curative treatment, the oncologist continues to check on J.S. to reassure her that she is not being abandoned.

J.S. is hospitalized 15 times over a period of 18 months for pain control, shortness of breath, infection, pleural effusion, small bowel obstruction, leptomeningeal disease, and shunt adjustments. She receives 14 consults, including neurology/neurosurgery, gastrointestinal, pulmonary, nutrition, psychology, psychiatry, rehabilitation, and radiation oncology, as well as 15 chaplaincy contacts. She refuses any discussion of hospice.

On the evening before her death, she is admitted for pain control and shortness of breath with full code status. Palliative care is called immediately, with a special request for the chaplain. Four hours before she dies, J.S.'s husband agrees to make her status do not resuscitate.

Eighteen months after her initial diagnosis, J.S. dies in the intensive care unit with an altered level of consciousness, shortness of breath, terminal delirium, and intractable pain.

## Summary and Key Points

Not every case has a tidy ending. Even if everything is done correctly, sometimes patients still suffer. J.S. and her husband could not bring themselves to verbalize the severity of J.S.'s cancer, which made it almost impossible to effectively control her pain and symptoms. She refused several hospitalizations and blood transfusions, wanting rather to go home. J.S. and her husband refused to let themselves or anyone else talk about her condition to their children. The team was exhausted.

The chaplain built a rapport with J.S. and her husband. He met alone with the husband several times, providing a safe outlet to share and vent feelings. During a visit close to J.S.'s death, the couple shared with the chaplain their anger at God. They were trying desperately to cling to hope. The chaplain discussed their issues at length. Before leaving, J.S. and her husband requested prayer. All involved with this case felt the blow of J.S.'s death. From the beginning, everyone had worked together to navigate holistic care for her.

- Early involvement of palliative care with concurrent treatment can improve quality of life.
- Palliative care teams work concurrently with the treating physician and nurse.
- As described by the National Consensus Project for Quality Palliative Care (2016), "The goal of palliative care is to prevent and relieve suffering to support the best possible quality of life for patients and their families, regardless of the stage of the disease or the need for other therapies . . . As such, it can be delivered concurrently with life-prolonging care or as the main focus of care."
- Family conferences are opportunities for open communication. They offer family care that is integrated, interactive, and inclusive (Fineberg & Bauer, 2011).
- Providing spiritual care is an important component of cancer care.
- Chaplains are trained to take in-depth spiritual histories, enabling them to address spiritual distress, support religious and spiritual resources, encourage spiritual coping, and resolve

spiritual problems (Sinclair & Chochinov, 2012; VandeCreek & Burton, 2001).

- Unfortunately, addressing spiritual concerns often is put off until closer to the end of life. It is important to address these concerns closer to the time of diagnosis, as it may facilitate adjustment throughout the illness trajectory (National Cancer Institute, 2015).

# Questions

## Why is it important to provide palliative care concurrently with cancer treatment?

Research has shown that involving palliative care early in the cancer diagnosis can improve quality of life and mitigate symptoms (Bakitas et al., 2009).

## Why is addressing the patient's spirituality vital to whole-person cancer care?

Research has shown that patients diagnosed with a terminal illness think about spirituality as a major factor in their quality of life (Taylor, 2015). Chaplains are well trained to address spiritual issues.

# References

Bakitas, M., Lyons, K.D., Hegel, M.T., Balan, S., Brokaw, F.C., Seville, J., … Ahles, T.A. (2009). Effects of a palliative care intervention on clinical outcomes in patients with advanced cancer: The Project ENABLE II randomized controlled trial. *JAMA, 302,* 741–749. doi:10.1001/jama.2009.1198

Child Life Council. (n.d.). The child life profession. Retrieved from http://www.childlife.org/The%20Child%20Life%20Profession

Dahlin, C. (Ed.). (2013). *Clinical practice guidelines for quality palliative care* (3rd ed.). Pittsburgh, PA: National Consensus Project for Quality Palliative Care.

Fineberg, I.C., & Bauer, A. (2011). Families and family conferencing. In T. Altilio & S. Otis-Green (Eds.), *Oxford textbook of palliative social work* (pp. 235–249). New York, NY: Oxford University Press.

National Cancer Institute. (2015). Spirituality in cancer care (PDQ®) [Patient version]. Retrieved from http://www.cancer.gov/about-cancer/coping/day-to-day/faith-and-spirituality/spirituality-pdq#section/_1

National Consensus Project for Quality Palliative Care. (2016). What is palliative care? Retrieved from http://www.nationalconsensusproject.org/DisplayPage.aspx?Title=What%20Is%20Palliative%20Care?

Puchalski, C., & Ferrell, B. (2010). *Making health care whole: Integrating spirituality into patient care.* West Conshohocken, PA: Templeton Press.

Sinclair, S., & Chochinov, H.M. (2012). The role of chaplains within oncology interdisciplinary teams. *Current Opinion in Supportive and Palliative Care, 6,* 259–268. doi:10.1097/SPC.0b013e3283521ec9

Taylor, E.J. (2015). Spiritual assessment. In B.R. Ferrell, N. Coyle, & J. Paice (Eds.), *Oxford textbook of palliative nursing* (4th ed., pp. 531–545). New York, NY: Oxford University Press.

Temel, J.S., Greer, J.A., Muzikansky, A., Gallagher, E.R., Admane, S., Jackson, V.A., … Lynch, T.J. (2010). Early palliative care for patients with metastatic non–small-cell lung cancer. *New England Journal of Medicine, 363,* 733–742. doi:10.1056/NEJMoa1000678

VandeCreek, L., & Burton, L. (2001). *Professional chaplain: Its role and importance in healthcare* [White paper]. Retrieved from http://www.healthcarechaplaincy.org/userimages/professional-chaplaincy-its-role-and-importance-in-healthcare.pdf

# The Post-Treatment Phase

Anne Zobec, MS, AOCNP®, BC, and Elissa A. Peters, RN, MS, OCN®, CBCN®

H.M. is a 45-year-old married woman with two school-aged children. She works full-time as an RN. H.M. also is a breast cancer survivor. She recently finished treatment for stage IIA triple-negative breast cancer, which included neoadjuvant chemotherapy, a bilateral mastectomy with sentinel lymph node biopsy and immediate reconstruction, and radiation. H.M. has no family history of cancer, but she did have genetic counseling and genetic testing; she tested negative for any genetic mutations.

## What is the role of the oncology nurse navigator (ONN) in communicating post-treatment support for a breast cancer diagnosis?

H.M. is followed by a disease-specific nurse navigator throughout her treatment and post-treatment. The ONN communicates with H.M. through office visits, during chemotherapy infusions, and over the phone.

On the last day of H.M.'s radiation treatment, the ONN meets briefly with her. Because they have established a therapeutic relationship during the course of her diagnosis and treatment, H.M. is comfortable confiding in her ONN. During this brief encounter, H.M. states mixed feelings about finishing her treatment. She feels she has more questions and concerns now that treatment is complete. Her questions include the following:

- How do I manage ongoing fatigue and other lingering side effects from treatment?

- How often do I see my oncologist now?
- How do I know if the cancer is gone?
- What if the cancer comes back?

The ONN asks H.M. more about her questions and concerns. H.M. believes she still needs to see her plastic surgeon to complete the tissue expansion and final implant exchange for her immediate breast reconstruction. Although she has not had any skin issues with her radiation treatment, H.M. is anxious that she still could have problems with her implants. She is aware that radiation can be a risk factor for breast implant failure. During active treatment, she was able to take a leave of absence from her job. Now that treatment is complete, H.M. really would like to get back to work; however, she feels so tired in the afternoons. H.M. is concerned about being able to mentally and physically keep up at work. She claims that she is unable to multitask like she used to.

H.M. complains that her fingernails are brittle and is worried that they will fall off. She also has lingering peripheral neuropathy that affects her fine motor skills. H.M. claims the numbness and tingling in her hands and feet seem to be less bothersome as she gets further from her last round of chemotherapy, but they still are present. H.M. has difficulty with tasks such as buttoning her clothes and cutting fruits and vegetables. Coupled with fatigue, this has her quite concerned about returning to work. As for her home life, H.M.'s husband and two children have been very supportive with household chores. She expresses concern that her family will want her to take over the household duties again, even though she feels so tired. H.M. is excited that her hair has started to grow back; however, she has received comments from her friends and family that concern her. H.M.'s husband, in particular, has mentioned that she must feel better because she "looks" better, and H.M. does not know how to explain that she is still feeling fatigued from treatment.

H.M. admits to not sleeping well and feeling overwhelmed when she lies down for the night. She is concerned about her diet and wants to cut out all sugars. She did not pay a lot of attention to her eating habits while on treatment, stating, "I just ate whatever sounded good at the time."

Emotional support and active listening are used when the ONN visits with H.M. The ONN assures H.M. that her questions and concerns are common for someone who has completed the acute portion of treatment.

## How can the ONN provide education and guidance on H.M.'s personal survivorship plan of care?

In previous meetings, the ONN talked with H.M. about post-treatment care and reinforced information surrounding the importance of a follow-up care plan. Now the ONN offers to make an appointment with her medical oncologist's office for a post-treatment survivorship visit; H.M. agrees. The ONN also refers the patient to a dietitian and oncology social worker. Once the survivorship visit is scheduled, the ONN discusses the case with a nurse practitioner (NP) to assess the need for physical therapy for H.M.'s cancer-related fatigue. As a key part of the multidisciplinary team, the ONN ensures that the patient's individual needs are met and assists in facilitation of referrals, ensuring that the patient does not "fall through the cracks" in post-treatment care.

## What is the role of the ONN as part of the multidisciplinary team?

At the post-treatment survivorship visit with the oncologist's NP, H.M. is able to spend a full hour discussing her concerns. The visit starts with H.M. sharing the story of her cancer journey with the NP. Although the NP has worked with her throughout her treatment and knows the clinical situation, H.M. finds it helpful to tell her story. The ONN completes a personal treatment summary and a personalized follow-up care plan for H.M. The plan is reviewed in detail with H.M. The NP is able to explain H.M.'s follow-up plan for the next 5–10 years, which H.M. finds very helpful.

H.M. did not attend any support groups while going through treatment, but she shows interest now that it is completed. She starts by attending a yoga class offered at the cancer center. Here, she meets other women in similar situations. She no longer feels as if she is the only one fearful of recurrence. Not only does she benefit from the group setting, but she also starts to use the breathing exercises she learns in class when feeling stressed at home.

H.M. admits that she and her husband have not made love since her breast cancer diagnosis. Initially, she felt very uncomfortable with the side effects of chemotherapy (Katz, 2009). She always felt "exhausted" and did not have time or energy to be intimate with her husband. After her mastectomy, she could not tolerate hugging or close body contact.

It has been so long since H.M. has been intimate that she feels "strange" and does not know how to initiate lovemaking. Her husband has been more tense and irritable. He expresses feelings of being overwhelmed with working, caring for the kids, and "keeping everything going" during H.M.'s illness. The NP gives H.M. a booklet on understanding intimacy and sexuality. H.M. is anxious to read it and hopes she will find some helpful information.

H.M. also is experiencing intense hot flashes—both day and night—and is waking multiple times during the night. This seems to have added to her fatigue, making H.M. feel irritable and unhappy. With a total lack of body hair, her breast surgery changes, and the emotional upheaval of menopause symptoms, she does not feel very attractive. As many as 50%–90% of survivors of breast cancer report concerns about sexual health. Nearly a third of these women may have problems lasting for many years (Cavallo, 2016).

H.M. is encouraged to gradually incorporate touch with her husband (e.g., caressing his arm, giving a quick hug, rubbing his back). H.M. also is advised to expand her ideas about intimacy and to not limit sex to the act of intercourse. Hugging, massaging, cuddling, and kissing can be very satisfying both physically and emotionally. If H.M. and her husband feel comfortable enough, oral sex also might be an option. The NP recommends that H.M. use vaginal lubricants and moisturizers to minimize dryness. H.M. is given some samples and a list of products she can find at a store or online.

The NP also suggests a selective serotonin reuptake inhibitor to minimize hot flashes, reduce night sweats, and improve sleep. This medication is helpful, and H.M.'s hot flashes are reduced by about 50%. Consequently, H.M. feels rested and has a bit more energy.

H.M. and her husband go on a "date night" and gently discuss the concerns about their sex life. She advises her husband that she wants to take things slowly. He appreciates her willingness to talk about this tough subject. They determine that the goal of their lovemaking will be to have pleasure—rather than intercourse—until they feel more comfortable and can better judge how H.M.'s body is responding.

Together, the ONN and the NP make suggestions to H.M. on how to get her health back on track, including the following:

1. Place your needs first. Try to do things you enjoy and that make you feel emotionally healthier.

2.  Eat a well-balanced diet.
3.  Begin a regular exercise program.

H.M. takes their advice and puts her needs first. She schedules and has a very productive meeting with the dietitian. For exercise, a neighbor agrees to be H.M.'s "buddy" for daily walks. At this point, H.M. achieves a more positive perspective on her personal survivorship plan.

## Summary and Key Points

H.M., a young, active woman, recently completed treatment for breast cancer. She is a wife, mom, friend, daughter, and RN. H.M. faced many challenges during treatment and will face many more in her breast cancer survivorship. The ONN and NP assisted her transition from patient to survivor, using their roles to individualize her care every step of the way.

- Patients need support in their transition to the post-treatment phase of the illness trajectory. This support can be multidisciplinary in nature and should be individualized to each patient.
- Fatigue, nail changes, peripheral neuropathy, insomnia, anxiety, fear of recurrence, sexual health, and body image concerns are common for young women with breast cancer who have received chemotherapy, breast surgery, and radiation. All can have a significant impact on quality of life following treatment.
- It can be helpful to assist these patients in setting goals for the next phase in their cancer journey.

## Questions

### When discussing the long-term implications of chemotherapy-induced peripheral neuropathy, what key points should the ONN and NP keep in mind?

Peripheral neuropathy can cause distress for patients trying to care for a family and work in a hands-on occupation. It can be painful, affect sleep quality, cause dexterity changes, and affect ambulation. Tingling and numbness can be a safety issue, as patients may be unable to feel temperature changes and may have difficulty walking (Smith & Zanville, 2015). No current evidence-based interventions exist to prevent or reduce peripheral neuropathy with cancer treatment. Duloxetine may be effective for pain and peripheral neuropathy. It is important to educate patients to communicate signs and symptoms early with their providers, teach safety strategies and proper foot care, and discuss strategies to prevent autonomic dysfunction (Tofthagen et al., 2015).

## What are the most common sexual problems for women after cancer treatment?

The most common problems for women include loss of sexual desire, hot flashes, night sweats, vaginal dryness and tightness, and pain with sex (Cavallo, 2016).

## What services should be provided to address sexual dysfunction after cancer?

Most problems with sexual dysfunction involve an organic deficit as well as the emotions of sexual dysfunction. Optimal programs combine gynecologic and urologic consultation with counseling by a mental health professional trained in both psycho-oncology and sex therapy (Miller, 2010).

## What are the major concerns for survivors of cancer?

The top five concerns for cancer survivors are fear of recurrence, fatigue, living with uncertainty, managing stress, and sleep disturbance (Ness et al., 2013).

## Why do nurses fail to discuss sexual concerns with their patients?

Nurses may feel that they have a lack of knowledge and limited resources to provide their patients. They also may have some discomfort with such a sensitive topic (Katz, 2009, 2016).

## References

Cavallo, J. (2016). *Guide to understanding intimacy and sexuality* (3rd ed.) [Pamphlet]. Retrieved from http://www.lbbc.org/intimacyguide

Katz, A. (2009). *Woman cancer sex*. Pittsburgh, PA: Hygeia Media.

Katz, A. (2016). Providing care for the whole patient: Sexuality and cancer. *Oncology Nurse-APN/PA, 9*(2), 6.

Miller, K.D. (Ed.). (2010). *Medical and psychosocial care of the cancer survivor.* Burlington, MA: Jones & Bartlett Learning.

Ness, S., Kokal, J., Fee-Schroeder, K., Novotny, P., Satele, D., & Barton, D. (2013). Concerns across the survivorship trajectory: Results from a survey of cancer survivors. *Oncology Nursing Forum, 40,* 35–42. doi:10.1188/13.ONF.35-42

Smith, E.M., & Zanville, N. (2015). Peripheral neuropathy. In C.G. Brown (Ed.), *A guide to oncology symptom management* (2nd ed., pp. 531–549). Pittsburgh, PA: Oncology Nursing Society.

Tofthagen, C.S., Visovsky, C., Camp-Sorrell, D., Collins, M.L., Erb, C.H., Olson, E.K., & Wood, S.K. (2015). Putting evidence into practice: Peripheral neuropathy. Retrieved from https://www.ons.org/practice-resources/pep/peripheral-neuropathy

# The Unexpected Caregiver

Eleanor Miller, MSN, RN, OCN®, CBCN®

S.G. is a 56-year-old man who works as a school administrator. At a school picnic, he develops difficulty with his speech. A trip to the emergency department (ED) and a computed tomography scan of his head reveals a lesion in his brain. A biopsy confirms a glioblastoma.

S.G. is referred to an oncology nurse navigator (ONN) to facilitate outpatient consults on discharge and offer overall support. S.G.'s main caregiver is his girlfriend. S.G.'s girlfriend explains that she and S.G. are not married and have been together for less than a year. However, she believes that they are in a place in their relationship where she would feel comfortable tending to S.G. as a caregiver.

## How should the ONN support S.G.'s caregivers?

The ONN should assess caregiver and patient needs with the following questions:
- Who is the main caregiver (e.g., significant other, parent, child, spouse, sibling, friend)?
- Who makes the decisions? Is this documented?
- How is it going at home? Is the patient independent or does he rely on others for assistance?
- What physical needs exist (e.g., bathing, dressing, walking)? Is a caregiver able to help with these physical needs?
- What emotional needs exist? Assess caregivers' emotions and their need for general emotional support, counseling, or respite (Skalla, Smith, Li, & Gates, 2013).
- Are the caregivers sleeping and eating properly?

- Who else is available to help? What family, friends, neighbors, coworkers, or church members are around for assistance?
- What type of employment do the patient and caregivers have? What are the sources of household income?
- Do specific transportation needs exist?
- What is helpful for the patient or caregivers in times of stress? Do they have informal and formal support? Value is found in both.
- What healthy activities are available (e.g., exercise, leisure time, reading, attending activities)?
- What education is needed? This needs to be continually revisited, focusing on both patient and caregiver education.
- What follow-up appointments are needed? It is best to plan ahead and keep things organized.
- A supportive ONN should allow the patient and caregivers the chance to sort through and solve any problems.

## What does the ONN need to know about S.G.'s family dynamic?

S.G. lives a great distance from the cancer center where he had surgery. It is recommended that he get radiation locally. This will ease the burden of getting to treatment. S.G. also is recommended to receive oral chemotherapy, which has a specific schedule.

S.G. has local family support. His 25-year-old daughter acts as his power of attorney. She signs the consent forms for his oral chemotherapy, as he is not able to do so himself. His girlfriend still is his main caregiver and continues to work as a full-time manager for a local department store. She works evenings, allowing her to attend S.G.'s daytime appointments prior to work. She notes feeling fatigued and overwhelmed; however, she is eager to participate in S.G.'s care.

## What interventions can the ONN suggest based on assessment of the family dynamic?

- Education: Teach information about the disease, medications, nutrition, and ideas for how to get everything accomplished. Educate on the difference between hospice and palliative care (Bevans et al., 2016).

- Communication: Facilitate answers to questions for patients and their families, including the following:
  - What is the medication schedule?
  - What is the plan if a certain treatment is pursued?
  - When are the next scans?
  - What appointments are needed?
  - Which appointments can be skipped?
  - Who is the contact for various needs?
  - What does the patient want or desire?
- Advocacy: Help by speaking on behalf of the patient, especially if it comes to discussing a realistic plan, end-of-life goals, or other important issues such as the following:
  - Does it make sense to drive a far distance if treatment is locally available?
  - What does insurance cover?
  - How do covered services integrate with treatment plans or recommendations?
  - What does recovery from surgery look like?
- Referral: Provide referrals for the patient and caregivers to other specialists and supportive services, including financial counselors, social workers, therapists, support groups, and other healthcare providers (Bevans et al., 2016; Rivera, 2009; Skalla et al., 2013).
- Emotional support: Give the caregivers credit! Remind them how lucky the patient is to have them and that they are doing a great job. Acknowledge the stress they are under and validate any emotions. Give them permission to speak and feel whatever they are feeling. They will probably feel guilty for being tired, stressed, or angry. Praise their commitment and focus (Bevans et al., 2016).
- Collaboration: Brainstorm ideas with the caregivers about how to best help the patient. They need to collaborate with the ONN, the medical team, and anyone else involved in patient care.

## How can the ONN assist in coordination of care?

Appointments with medical and radiation oncology are scheduled soon after S.G.'s discharge. He will arrive at his appointments by ambulance, as he still is not able to walk postsurgery. Following these appointments, education is provided to S.G.'s family and his girlfriend about the chemotherapy and radiation plan as well as resources that will be put into place after S.G.'s discharge from rehabilitation. Referrals are made to the ONN at his local cancer center to schedule consultations with local oncologists. The ONN's role also is emphasized as an extra layer of support to the patient and caregivers. It is suggested that S.G.'s family and girlfriend access counseling to sort out emotions after the diagnosis. Financial resources are not a major concern because of the disability benefit provided through S.G.'s employer. These conversations are communicated with the entire care team.

## Summary and Key Points

S.G. is a man facing an unexpected life-threatening illness. After his diagnosis, S.G.'s new girlfriend decided to serve as his main caregiver. She was scared, hopeful, and overwhelmed, but she also was focused. It was paramount to reassure S.G.'s girlfriend and his daughter that they could call their ONN for help with education, support, or appointments.

Support was evident when S.G.'s girlfriend forgot some of the discharge instructions and called the ONN for help. She also called to clarify the steroid taper schedule. Once initial needs were met, the ONN made sure to acknowledge her role, encourage her, and check on her well-being. It was important to assess the big picture with S.G.'s girlfriend, enabling her to have a clear understanding of the future.

S.G. and his girlfriend will be back to meet with a medical oncologist and a neurosurgeon. When the time comes, the ONN and S.G.'s medical team will have a conversation with his girlfriend about his end-of-life care. That conversation will not be easy, but the ONN, who has worked with S.G.'s girlfriend throughout this journey, will be able to help her cope when the time comes. Family dynamics and caregivers provide unique, surprising challenges for an ONN.

- An ONN can help ensure smooth care transitions into a community where providers often are less familiar with complex oncology cases and the needs of these patients and their caregivers.
- An ONN can provide support for team members and education about the disease and plan of care.
- A report on caregiving in the United States revealed that 43.5 million adults served as unpaid caregivers in 2015. On average, these caregivers provided 24.4 hours of care per week, while some provided 40 or more hours of care (National Alliance for Caregiving & AARP Public Policy Institute, 2015).

- Many needs and concerns exist for caregivers, including fatigue and depression (Rivera, 2009; Skalla et al., 2013; Whisenant, 2011). Caregivers could run away from the situation (and might want to at times), but they show commitment, unconditional love, and loyalty in extraordinary ways.
- Brain tumors generally comprise about 2% of all newly diagnosed adult cancers (Dolinsky, Millar, & Vachani, 2015).
- In 2016, an estimated 78,000 new cases of primary brain tumors, both benign (53,000) and malignant (25,000), were diagnosed in the United States (American Brain Tumor Association, 2014). The peak age for diagnosis varies with tumor type; however, when accounting for all types, the average age is about 50 years (Dolinsky et al., 2015).
- Diagnosis of brain tumors is done by magnetic resonance imaging (MRI). A contrast of the brain is used to evaluate whether a tumor is present and to characterize it.
- Although imaging is suggestive of a brain tumor, the type of brain tumor cannot be known until a biopsy is done and a tissue sample is sent to pathology for confirmation.
- All caregivers need education and support, but some caregivers might need a bit more encouragement, motivation, and credit, as they are in this role out of unconditional love.
- ONNs only know their patients for a short time. Caregivers can give much-needed and detailed insight on patients and provide physical and emotional care.
- Without caregivers, many patients would remain in the hospital or other facilities. Caregivers help patients to be able to live at home (Skalla et al., 2013).
- Caregiving is a demonstration of commitment, strength, and courage. The role can sometimes be emotional, stressful, anxiety provoking, overwhelming, or scary.
- Regardless of the relationship, caregivers experience many needs in their role, including physical, emotional, financial, and spiritual issues. These can be addressed by an ONN.

## Questions

### When S.G. has a repeat MRI and it shows progression, how should the ONN proceed?

First, the ONN should communicate the next steps to the team and coordinate the logistics of the plan with S.G.'s family. The ONN should determine if S.G. needs a referral back to neurosurgery or return visits with medical or radiation oncology. If S.G. is interested or eligible, the ONN then could coordinate an evaluation for a clinical trial (Bevans et al., 2016).

### If S.G.'s girlfriend expresses exhaustion and is short tempered, what resources should the ONN suggest?

The ONN should offer emotional support to see if S.G.'s girlfriend is self-aware of her condition or if it needs to be acknowledged. The ONN could make referrals for respite or support groups, or tap into additional homecare or family resources (Rivera, 2009; Skalla et al., 2013; Whisenant, 2011).

## References

American Brain Tumor Association. (2014). Brain tumor statistics. Retrieved from http://www.abta.org/about-us/news/brain-tumor-statistics

Bevans, M.F., Cagle, C.S., Coleman, M., Haisfield-Wolfe, M.E., Jadalla, A., Page, M., & Sundaramurthi, T. (2016). Putting evidence into practice: Caregiver strain and burden. Retrieved from https://www.ons.org/practice-resources/pep/caregiver -strain-and-burden

Dolinsky, C., Millar, L.B., & Vachani, C. (2015). All about brain tumors. Retrieved from https://www.oncolink.org/types/article.cfm?c=52&aid=247&id=9534

National Alliance for Caregiving & AARP Public Policy Institute. (2015). *Caregiving in the U.S.: Executive summary*. Retrieved from http://www.caregiving.org/wp-content/ uploads/2015/05/2015_CaregivingintheUS_Executive-Summary-June -4_WEB.pdf

Rivera, H.R. (2009). Depression symptoms in cancer caregivers. *Clinical Journal of Oncology Nursing, 13*, 195–202. doi:10.1188/09.CJON.195-202

Skalla, K.A., Smith, E.M.L., Li, Z., & Gates, C. (2013). Multidimensional needs of caregivers for patients with cancer. *Clinical Journal of Oncology Nursing, 17*, 500– 506. doi:10.1188/13.CJON.17-05AP

Whisenant, M. (2011). Informal caregiving in patients with brain tumors [Online exclusive]. *Oncology Nursing Forum, 38*, E373–E381. doi:10.1188/11.ONF. E373-E381

# Navigator Collaboration

Amy Sebastian-Deutsch, DNP, APRN, CNS, AOCNS®

The partnership of a professional navigator with a lay navigator (LN) can be very powerful in knocking down barriers to care that frequently result in treatment delays. The following examples of partnerships with positive patient outcomes are from a Houston, Texas, navigator chapter.

In one example, a Latino patient with cancer was referred by an oncology nurse navigator (ONN) to an LN for help with finding financial assistance to cover the costs of care. The LN found that the patient qualified for county funds designated for Spanish-speaking patients in need of treatment. The ONN had not been aware of this resource.

In another example, an LN from a local community center contacted an ONN regarding a patient with cancer who needed assistance with nutrition. The ONN enrolled the patient into a free dietary program provided by her hospital. There, the patient received nutrition education and was assessed for malnutrition by the hospital's dietitian. The patient also was confused about her appointments and what was going to happen in the future. The LN discussed the patient's fears with the ONN. To help alleviate the patient's anxiety, the LN requested that the ONN contact the patient and explain the plan of care.

As a final example, a patient lost her insurance coverage during the middle of treatment. The ONN contacted the LN at another local treatment center. The LN was able to facilitate the transfer of care, ensuring an optimal patient outcome.

These short scenarios detail the importance of daily collaboration on a one-to-one level between two different types of navigators and the positive outcomes experienced by the patients they conavigated.

## What are the roles of the ONN and LN?

In the field of oncology, patient navigation within the hospital setting is generally carried out by an ONN, as opposed to an LN. The Oncology Nursing Society's (ONS's) *Oncology Nurse Navigator Core Competencies* provide two definitions to differentiate between the professional versus lay navigator (ONS, 2013).

The ONN is "a professional RN with oncology-specific clinical knowledge who offers individualized assistance to patients, families, and caregivers to help overcome healthcare system barriers. Using the nursing process, an ONN provides education and resources to facilitate informed decision making and timely access to quality health and psychosocial care throughout all phases of the cancer continuum" (ONS, 2013, p. 6).

The LN is "a trained nonprofessional or volunteer who provides individualized assistance to patients, families, and caregivers to help overcome healthcare system barriers and facilitate timely access to quality health and psychosocial care from prediagnosis through all phases of the cancer experience" (ONS, 2013, p. 6).

The LN is not a paid professional and does not generally work in the hospital but may work within the local community. According to the Academy of Oncology Nurse and Patient Navigators (AONN, n.d.), a layperson can be a navigator. The role of this person is to "fulfill specific administrative tasks to expedite scheduling or access to resources, and carry out other functions appropriate for a nonmedical person to perform" (AONN, n.d., para. 3).

## How is collaboration defined in patient navigation?

According to the Association for Information and Image Management (AIIM), "Collaboration enables individuals to work together to achieve a defined and common business purpose" (AIIM, n.d.). AIIM also indicates that collaboration relies on the ability of people to be open and the willingness to share knowledge while maintaining some level of focus and responsibility. In patient navigation, collaboration enables the licensed navigator (the ONN) and the unlicensed patient navigator (the LN or community health worker) to openly and willingly share knowledge about resources and treatment strategies to overcome barriers to care for patients with cancer. Collaboration also helps to achieve the best possible outcomes for those needing navigation.

During the provision of care for patients with cancer, the roles of ONNs and LNs often intersect on a daily basis; however, collaboration between oncology navigators (professional and lay) also can happen on a much larger scale.

A chapter of AONN recently was formed in Houston, Texas. This chapter is led by A.S., an ONN who works at a large local health system. A.S. and a group of nine ONNs from the health system have been meeting internally to share best practices and pool their resources. A.S. wants to expand their network, so forming a local chapter seems like the next logical step.

Soon after creating this new chapter, membership increases to 17 members representing four organizations. Officers are elected at the first meeting, and membership now includes LNs with additional organizations represented. A.S. also shares her vision for the future of the local chapter. She hopes to grow the membership to include community health workers and a central repository where community resources can be accessible to all chapter members.

Her vision for the chapter is to build partnerships among local ONNs and other oncology patient navigators. She hopes to incorporate their shared knowledge, expertise, resources, networking, and education to help meet the needs of locally served patients and survivors.

With this vision in mind, A.S. desires to develop a Houston central repository that includes helpful resources for both LNs and professional navigators. The repository would need to be accessible by all chapter members for use by the people they navigate. In a rather fortuitous turn of events, a chapter member, S.B., hears about a new product called Journey Connections (Lilly Oncology, n.d.).

S.B. explains how Journey Connections would allow for the upload of local navigator resources into a database. Based on assessed individual patient needs, the database could be searched by category, then a page of resources could be printed for the patient.

A.S. likes the idea so much she suggests a formal presentation on the product at a future chapter meeting. The chapter members (both ONNs and LNs) are in agreement and a presentation is arranged. Key presentation points include the following:

- **The need**—Patients diagnosed with cancer have many needs, including medical, emotional, informational, and practical needs. They need help from a trusted individual.

- **The solution**—Journey Connections provides a way for navigators to provide support for their patients by accessing a printable list of local resources based on their assessed needs (Lilly Oncology, n.d.).
- **The benefits**—Journey Connections provides a way to organize and customize patient support resources and quickly and efficiently deliver information to patients in a standardized format (Lilly Oncology, n.d.).

The database is built around 12 categories and includes an interactive map showing locations of beneficial local businesses for patients:

1. Accessories
2. Emotional support
3. Financial assistance
4. Food and nutrition
5. Home and family care
6. Hospice and respite
7. Legal assistance
8. Medical services
9. Physical well-being
10. Programs and events
11. Transportation
12. Wish fulfillment

Chapter members submit their lists of resources on a template to S.B., now the Journey Connections coordinator. She enters the resources into the database. Once these data are entered, each navigator can either print or download a personalized handout for each patient.

This exemplar defines what can be achieved when people are willing to share ideas and resources. In this case, it is through the collaborative efforts of ONNs, LNs, and healthcare teams. Houston is a city of about four million people. The potential benefit of this collaboration to the general population could be staggering. The sheer scope of this collaboration can only serve to benefit existing patients and will most assuredly assist future patients with cancer within the Houston area.

## Summary and Key Points

This chapter described the benefits of combining the skills of LNs and ONNs through small case studies and collaborative efforts.

Through collaboration, the ONN and LN are able to work together to achieve a defined and common navigation purpose, knock down barriers to care, and minimize treatment delays.
- By joining forces, professional and lay navigators can overcome many barriers that they may not be able to individually resolve.
- Never underestimate the power of collaboration.

## Questions

**Within the hospital setting, the ONN generally is an RN with what type of experience?**

The ONN typically has oncology-specific knowledge and uses the nursing process to aid patients in informed decision making.

**What is the definition of collaboration in navigation?**

Effective ONNs should embrace collaboration. Collaboration in this instance is relying on the ability of people to be open and willing to share knowledge to achieve a common purpose: navigation of the patient.

## References

Academy of Oncology Nurse and Patient Navigators. (n.d.). Helpful definitions. Retrieved from https://www.aonnonline.org/about/helpful-definitions

Association for Information and Image Management. (n.d.). What is collaboration? Retrieved from http://www.aiim.org/What-is-Collaboration

Lilly Oncology. (n.d.). Journey Connections. Retrieved from http://www.lillyoncology.com/resources/journey-connections.html

Oncology Nursing Society. (2013). *Oncology nurse navigator core competencies.* Retrieved from https://www. ons.org/sites/default/files/ONNCompetencies_rev.pdf

## CASE 22
# Oncology Nurse Navigator Integration Into the Multidisciplinary Care Continuum

Emily Mason Beard, RN, BSN, OCN®, CBCN®

A.B. is a 37-year-old marathon runner who notices a tugging sensation along her right breast while exercising. Later, she feels a nontender lump in the same area. Three months ago, A.B. lost her job and health benefits when her company downsized. Consolidated Omnibus Budget Reconciliation Act (COBRA) premiums are too expensive, so she is without health insurance. A.B. is told she will have to wait several weeks to be added to her husband's health insurance policy. This causes severe anxiety for A.B., who was diagnosed with dense fibrocystic breast tissue at age 24 and has a history of a benign breast biopsy. She decides to pay out-of-pocket to see an obstetrician/gynecologist (OB/GYN). She is worried about the lump, but she also wants to discuss her unsuccessful attempts to get pregnant after trying for more than a year. The OB/GYN is very concerned about the breast lump and a second lump under A.B.'s arm, so he sends A.B. for a diagnostic mammogram and ultrasound.

### How can the unique role of the oncology nurse navigator (ONN) support a patient in the care continuum?

With ongoing changes in health care and a constantly evolving basis of evidence informing and individualizing cancer treatment recommendations, patients often are overwhelmed. ONNs are seasoned clinicians with valuable insights to assist patients with needs and barriers of all kinds, including physical, emotional, and practical.

A.B. panics when the technologist finishes her ultrasound and tells her a radiologist will be in to talk about the results. She wishes someone had come with her to the appointment. A.B. is comforted when the ONN for diagnostic services at the breast center enters the room, introduces herself, and tells A.B. that she will stay with her to provide support. The ONN is with A.B. when the radiologist explains that a biopsy is necessary, as A.B.'s mammogram and ultrasound are suspicious for breast cancer.

A.B. is very upset, fearful, and overwhelmed. She expected this lump to be benign and worries about the medical costs and her lack of insurance. The ONN stays with A.B. while she texts her husband and shares the news. A.B. cries so hard she can barely speak.

The ONN provides emotional support until A.B.'s husband can arrive. A.B. explains that she and her husband have only been married a year and that they really want to be parents. She already feels depressed about her inability to conceive and questions how she will deal with this new development.

The ONN schedules a biopsy for the next morning. In addition to explaining the biopsy procedure and instructions to A.B. and her husband, the ONN conducts a preprocedure physical assessment and arranges a meeting with a financial representative who can provide an estimate on cost. When A.B. leaves, she still is very anxious but also is relieved now that she knows what to expect. A.B.'s husband thanks the ONN for being a trustworthy and reliable guide.

## What is the ONN's role in a cancer diagnosis?

When patients fear that they might have a diagnosis of cancer, the distress only worsens the longer it takes to get a result. Given the defined categories of competency for the ONN role—professionalism, education, coordination, and communication—patients may be more willing to share personal struggles and needs with an ONN than with a physician or another member of the healthcare team (Oncology Nursing Society, 2013). That personal relationship builds trust and provides relevant insights into caring for the patient over time. Recognizing patients with complex psychosocial or physical situations who likely will need more support—emotional or physical—is of utmost importance. It is a role well-served by a diagnostic nurse navigator (Gilbert et al., 2011). To decrease anxiety and provide patient-centered care, ONNs are able to offer various services along the continuum, including assessment, education, support, and communication associated with waiting for results (Harding, 2015). In addition to support, ONNs coordinate ancillary services, including financial counseling and behavioral health services, to alleviate anxiety (Friedman et al., 2015).

## What is the purpose of the multidisciplinary care (MDC) continuum?

Physicians who treat cancer may have differing views about specific regimens and sequencing of treatment. Patients can get caught in the middle. For example, a surgeon might be eager to schedule a patient for surgery as a first step to resect a tumor, while the medical oncologist might prefer to initiate neoadjuvant chemotherapy in hopes that the tumor will shrink prior to operation. The conversation can be confusing to patients, especially if other barriers exist, such as language, low healthcare literacy, or anxiety. At its best, the MDC continuum approach draws the healthcare team together toward a consensus about treatment planning through "teamwork and synergistic patient care" (Hong, Gagliardi, Bronskill, Paszat, & Wright, 2010, p. 65); however, this approach does have drawbacks and can be overwhelming for newly diagnosed patients. MDC continuum delivery includes various settings and spans across many cancer care models (Fennel, Das, Clauser, Petrelli, & Salner, 2010).

The specifics of the navigation role vary dramatically from center to center, but the National Cancer Institute Community Cancer Centers Program described how oncology navigation programs generally fall into one of three models of MDC delivery (Swanson et al., 2012):

1. The cancer case conference or tumor board—In this model, members of the team meet privately to review the patient's imaging and pathology, discuss the diagnosis, and decide on treatment recommendations.
2. The dedicated disease site–specific clinic (e.g., thoracic, breast, gastrointestinal [GI], GYN)—In a site-specific clinic, patients consult with their primary team of specialists on the same day

and in the same location. Diagnostic results and follow-up care are coordinated on-site, often by an ONN.

3. The virtual clinic model—In this model, patients see their providers in separately scheduled appointments, which could be on the same day or over the course of weeks. Care is arranged by a central coordinator, which could be an ONN or other navigator.

A.B.'s pathology report comes back positive for invasive ductal cancer, strongly estrogen and progesterone receptor positive, and HER2 negative (1+). At 3.5 cm and with one positive lymph node, this is T2 N1 Mx, stage IIIA breast cancer. The radiologist notifies the ONN then calls A.B. with the news.

## How can the ONN facilitate coordination of care?

The ONN facilitates a next-day referral to the breast surgeon, based on the recommendation by A.B.'s OB/GYN. She verifies that the surgeon is able to accept self-pay patients and calls the oncology social worker to notify him of A.B.'s diagnosis and lack of insurance and financial resources. Based on the American Joint Committee on Cancer and National Comprehensive Cancer Network® (NCCN®) guidelines, the ONN understands that a cancer of this stage will require systemic and regional treatment with chemotherapy and surgery (NCCN, 2016b). She also calls the breast MDC clinic ONN for a report on A.B.'s diagnosis. The ONN regularly calls the clinic ONN about newly diagnosed patients who come through the clinic.

One of the main areas of competency for an ONN is care coordination. This is exemplified by both ONNs attending to the needs of their shared patient in a seamless and efficient manner. The clinic ONN is appreciative of the "heads up" from the ONN about some of A.B.'s unique concerns (e.g., lack of insurance, desire for fertility, high anxiety). This is the usual "handoff" process between the two ONNs. The clinic ONN is grateful to know what to expect when the patient arrives for her first visit.

At the end of the day, the ONN calls A.B. to check in with her, provide emotional support, confirm the time and location of her appointment with the surgeon, and ask if she has any questions or needs. She also tells A.B. that soon she will be meeting the clinic ONN, who will coordinate her care moving forward. She reassures A.B. that she will continue to be a resource.

## Is it necessary to have a separate ONN for each phase in the continuum of care?

The answer depends on the type of center, its structure, and case volume at hospitals. In some small community hospitals with relatively low volumes of patients, a single ONN might be able to facilitate the care of all the patients from diagnosis to treatment and beyond. This certainly is the easiest way, as there is no concern about patients getting lost between handoffs.

Some navigators may be disease-site specific (e.g., breast, thoracic, GI, GYN), whereas others may focus on one area of the continuum. For example, in larger centers, multiple diagnostic imaging navigators facilitating only the episode of care from diagnostic mammogram (or GI endoscopy or computed tomography lung screening) to biopsy may exist. These navigators then will hand off to a navigator who focuses on treatment planning after the pathologic diagnosis is confirmed. In many cancer centers, the ONN initiates patient care immediately after informing the patient of the diagnosis.

## How does the clinic ONN prepare for the needs of the newly diagnosed patient?

The clinic ONN adds A.B. to the schedule for the next breast cancer MDC clinic later in the week. The MDC model at this cancer center is a "virtual clinic," where weekly visits are made to individual physicians with care coordinated through the ONN.

The breast cancer MDC model allows the treatment team to develop plans and recommendations for treatment and to review imaging, pathology, and other relevant information about the patient's history. The clinic ONN coordinates all of these efforts, ensuring that the appropriate appointments and consultations are made.

Before she meets the patient, the clinic ONN develops a list of individualized priorities based on her knowledge of the diagnosis, stage, and appropriate treatment guidelines:

1. Referral to the genetic counselor—A.B. is under age 50; therefore, she should have a genetic evaluation based on national guidelines (NCCN, 2016c).

2. Referral from a medical oncologist for a reproductive endocrinologist—Systemic chemotherapy can cause irreversible gonadal failure in women of reproductive age. The clinic ONN knows to address fertility preservation options with the patient prior to initiation of chemotherapy (Loren et al., 2013).
3. Follow-up call to the oncology social worker regarding resources and insurance assistance—Multiple federal, state, and local resources can assist uninsured and underinsured patients in covering the costs of treatments.
4. Call to the clinical trial nurse regarding potential eligibility—NCCN guidelines recommend that all patients with cancer consider participating in clinical research as part of their treatment plan (NCCN, 2016c).
5. Gather information on local peer-to-peer support groups for young women with cancer—Young adult survivors often feel especially isolated and overwhelmed by their cancer diagnosis (NCCN, 2016a).

## How does the ONN enhance the MDC continuum?

A.B.'s case is presented to the weekly breast cancer MDC virtual clinic as follows:

> A.B. is a 37-year-old female recently diagnosed with stage IIIA invasive ductal breast cancer. She is married without children, but she desires pregnancy. A.B. otherwise is in excellent health, as she has no chronic health problems and enjoys hiking and competing in marathons. She first noticed a pulling sensation along her upper outer right breast. Weeks later, her OB/GYN palpated two hard, nonmobile lumps—one in her upper outer right breast and one in her axilla concerning for a lymph node. After a significant delay because of a job change and lack of insurance, A.B. presented at the diagnostic breast center for a mammogram and ultrasound.

At the virtual clinic, the radiologist reviews the initial mammogram and ultrasound, including the image-guided needle biopsy of the masses in the breast and axilla. The pathologist confirms a diagnosis of infiltrating ductal carcinoma, poorly differentiated. The surgeon then explains how he examined the patient and agreed that the tumor was "at least a T2."

Because of her age, the stage of her cancer, and her desire to have children, A.B. needs to visit a medical oncologist for consideration of neoadjuvant chemotherapy and discussion about fertility preservation. The clinic oncologist states that the patient actually is planning to undergo oocyte retrieval later in the week. The medical oncologist states that, even though she would have preferred for the patient to start chemotherapy immediately, it is reasonable to first address fertility concerns. The physicians agrees that A.B. should have a breast magnetic resonance imaging (MRI) scan prior to starting chemotherapy. The clinic ONN notes this recommendation and adds the order to her list of priorities for A.B. The clinical research team states that A.B. may be eligible to participate in a clinical trial. Once they collect more information from the MRI, the MDC team plans to present A.B.'s case again the following week.

## What is the clinic ONN's role as the patient progresses through treatment?

The clinic ONN's role is to assist in coordinating the patient's care and ensure that the patient has access to the guidance and support she will need to overcome various barriers to care.

At the time of A.B.'s diagnosis, the ONN anticipates certain common orders based on clinical guidelines, such as referral to the genetic counselor (given the patient's age of under 40 and, desire to preserve fertility, and the need for her to consult with a reproductive endocrinologist prior to initiation of chemotherapy). The ONN also alerts the oncology social worker to be on standby for psychosocial support and assistance with financial and insurance resources. She also expects certain imaging studies. The patient's hobbies, financial and insurance barriers, and overwhelming desire to preserve her fertility may seem insignificant compared to the overall seriousness of her cancer diagnosis, but these factors have a tremendous influence on the ONN's approach to treatment and decision making. Thanks to the clinic ONN's coordination efforts, A.B. is able to see a reproductive endocrinologist without much delay.

Two weeks after her biopsy, A.B. undergoes a procedure to harvest her eggs. She also sees a genetic counselor and is waiting to get her results. After working with them for two weeks, the oncology social worker gets in touch with A.B.'s husband's employer, advocating the employer to add A.B. to the insurance policy.

At a breast cancer MDC continuum two weeks later, the clinic ONN learns from the genetic counselor that A.B. has tested positive for a *BRCA1* mutation. A.B. is referred to a plastic surgeon to discuss options for breast reconstruction after mastectomy. The clinic ONN also learns that A.B. could qualify for a clinical trial based on her *BRCA* status.

A.B. completes her first cycle of chemotherapy. She is coping as well as she can and meets with her oncology social worker on each visit to address her anxiety, which is further exacerbated by her genetic testing results. With assistance from the social worker, A.B.'s husband's company agrees to cover A.B. under its insurance.

A.B.'s fertility preservation procedure is successful in retrieving oocytes, which results in eight fertilized embryos. A.B. is relieved and thanks the clinic ONN for ensuring that this step is completed. A.B. does not know if she will ever be able to use the embryos, but she is glad to have the option, as motherhood is one of her lifetime goals. She tells the clinic ONN that if her physician feels carrying a pregnancy is too risky, maybe she will use a gestational carrier. The clinic ONN will continue to check in with the patient and her husband throughout the continuum of care, as the patient completes chemotherapy, plans for surgery, and determines the need for radiation therapy.

At each transition of care, the MDC team will discuss her case. They will review her MRI after she completes chemotherapy and discuss her need for adjuvant radiation after her surgery and pathologic staging is complete. The clinic ONN will continue to monitor her care and record her treatment options and outcomes as she moves through the continuum.

## Summary and Key Points

In recent decades, quality cancer care delivery has become a complex process of facilitating shared decision making between the patient and multiple physicians. This care continuum often involves a team of specialists weighing in with a variety of diagnostic and treatment recommendations, which are individualized based on patient age, overall health, family history, stage of cancer, prognostic indicators, and other attributes of the cancer type. A prospective, patient-centered team planning model is supported by the National Academy of Medicine (formerly the Institute of Medicine) as an approach all cancer programs should strive to provide (Levit, Nass, & Ganz, 2013). Although the MDC is a standard of care in oncology, having so many providers to consult with can leave patients and their families feeling overwhelmed and frustrated. Breakdowns in communication can lead to fragmented care, knowledge gaps, decreased patient satisfaction, and potentially poor outcomes (Thorne, Bultz, & Baile, 2005). The addition of practical problems, such as insurance access, costs, underlying stress and anxiety, and cancer care, can be a burdensome maze through which to navigate for patients and their families. Nurses with specialty oncology training and skills in patient navigation have proven integral to the success of the multidisciplinary approach to care. The National Cancer Institute Community Cancer Centers Program found that having an experienced nurse navigator was a key factor for successful MDC program development in the community cancer center setting (Swanson et al., 2012). ONNs function as professional problem-solvers by identifying individual patient needs and coordinating appropriate support services that address barriers to care (Friedman et al., 2015). All patients with cancer are unique, having specific life experiences, goals, and priorities that shape their outlook on life and living with cancer. Personalizing care while adhering to standards and guidelines can be a challenge, requiring ongoing assessment, education, and communication. Although the ONN role still is relatively new, a growing evidence indicates that patient navigation is a critical part of the multidisciplinary team and the overall continuum of cancer care. Patients trust their nurses and are better satisfied knowing that they have a champion on their team—someone who is looking out for their best interests.

- The ONN is in a unique position along the care continuum, having the opportunity to develop trusting relationships with a patient from the start, improve understanding through communication, and decrease patient anxiety.
- Especially at times of uncertainty for the patient and family (e.g., prior to diagnosis, when test results are pending), the ONN can improve access and coordination of services.
- Cancers of all types are treated by multiple specialists, adding complexity to the treatment planning process.

- Depending on the type of healthcare system, MDC continuums can be structured in a variety of ways, but nurses and navigators play an important role.
- The ONN listens for information that may influence patient care while anticipating needs and plans for coordination of care.
- The ONN demonstrates knowledge of clinical guidelines by proactively identifying candidates for genetic testing, clinical research, and psychosocial support.
- The ONN recognizes needs and initiates timely referrals to other ancillary services.

## Questions

### Does the ONN need to have expertise in all areas of patient care, including barriers to care?

The ONN must have familiarity with community resources and specialty services, such as support groups, dietitians, physical therapists, and counselors with specialization in oncology. The ONN should seek and cultivate strong working relationships with various colleagues in the hospital, organization, or community who can act as resources for patients. The ONN can identify the needs of a particular patient and help provide individualized care through referral to ancillary services, including financial assistance, palliative care, physical and occupational rehabilitation, and behavioral health. This activity is most beneficial when these referrals and needs for services are communicated to the whole treatment team through participation and discussion in an MDC cancer conference or clinic meeting (Friedman et al., 2015).

### What is the best way for a nurse to prepare for a career as an ONN?

Because the ONN has such a critically important role in the overall success of a MDC program, it is important for an aspiring ONN to become familiar with the entire continuum of care—from screening and diagnosis to treatment and survivorship. It is helpful to job shadow in all areas where patients receive care to fully understand the continuum and the challenges that arise in each episode of a patient's care. Most nursing roles are specialized (e.g., interventional radiology, surgery, chemotherapy infusion, community health), making it important for a new ONN, even one seasoned in oncology, to learn about the less-familiar areas of the care continuum. A great way to begin developing the competencies for success as an ONN is to build relationships with other clinicians and members of the multidisciplinary team (e.g., physicians, physical therapists, dietitians, nurses in all areas of the care continuum). A new ONN could attend MDC continuums, educational grand rounds, quality committees, and community outreach activities. It is only with a solid background in all areas of oncology that a nurse can be a well-informed guide and care coordinator who can truly facilitate MDC and strong communication between specialists on a team (Swanson et al., 2012).

## References

Fennell, M.L., Das, I.P., Clauser, S., Petrelli, N., & Salner, A. (2010). The organization of multidisciplinary care teams: Modeling internal and external influences on cancer care quality. *Journal of the National Cancer Institute Monographs, 2010*(40), 72–80. doi:10.1093/jncimonographs/lgq010

Friedman, E.L., Chawla, N., Morris, P.T., Castro, K.M., Carrigan, A.C., Das, I.P., & Clauser, S.B. (2015). Assessing the development of multidisciplinary care: Experience of the National Cancer Institute Community Cancer Centers Program. *Journal of Oncology Practice, 11,* e36–e42. doi:10.1200/JOP.2014.001535

Gilbert, J.E., Green, E., Lankshear, S., Hughes, E., Burkoski, V., & Sawka, C. (2011). Nurses as patient navigators in cancer diagnosis: Review, consultation and model design. *European Journal of Cancer Care, 20,* 228–236. doi:10.1111/j.1365-2354.2010.01231.x

Harding, M. (2015). Effect of nurse navigation on patient care satisfaction and distress associated with breast biopsy [Online exclusive]. *Clinical Journal of Oncology Nursing, 19,* e15–e20. doi:10.1188/15.CJON.E15-E20

Hong, N.J.L., Gagliardi, A.R., Bronskill, S.E., Paszat, L.F., & Wright, F.C. (2010). Multidisciplinary cancer conferences: Exploring obstacles and facilitators to their implementation. *Journal of Oncology Practice, 6,* 61–68. doi:10.1200/JOP.091085

Levit, B.L., Nass, S., & Ganz, P.A. (Eds.). (2013). *Delivering high-quality cancer care: Charting a new course for a system in crisis.* Washington, DC: National Academies Press.

Loren, A.W., Mangu, P.B., Beck, L.N., Brennan, L., Magdalinski, A.J., Partridge, A.H., ... Oktay, K. (2013). Fertility preservation for patients with cancer: American Society of Clinical Oncology clinical practice guideline update. *Journal of Clinical Oncology, 31,* 2500–2510. doi:10.1200/jco.2013.49.2678

National Comprehensive Cancer Network. (2016a). *NCCN Clinical Practice Guidelines in Oncology (NCCN Guidelines®): Adolescent and young adult (AYA)* [v.1.2016]. Retrieved from http://www.nccn.org/professionals/physician_gls/pdf/aya.pdf

National Comprehensive Cancer Network. (2016b). *NCCN Clinical Practice Guidelines in Oncology (NCCN Guidelines®): Breast cancer* [v.2.2016]. Retrieved from https://www.nccn.org/professionals/physician_gls/pdf/breast.pdf

National Comprehensive Cancer Network. (2016c). *NCCN Clinical Practice Guidelines in Oncology (NCCN Guidelines®): Genetic/familial high-risk assessment: Breast and ovarian* [v.2.2016]. Retrieved from http://www.nccn.org/professionals/physician_gls/pdf/genetics_screening.pdf

Oncology Nursing Society. (2013). *Oncology nurse navigator core competencies.* Retrieved from https://www.ons.org/sites/default/files/ONNCompetencies_rev.pdf

Swanson, P.L., Strusowski, P., Asfeldt, T., De Groot, J., Hegedus, P.D., Krasna, M., & White, D. (2012, January/February). Expanding multidisciplinary care in community cancer centers: An MDC assessment tool developed by the NCCCP. *Oncology Issues,* pp. 33–37.

Thorne, S.E., Bultz, B.D., & Baile, W.F. (2005). Is there a cost to poor communication in cancer care? A critical review of the literature. *Psycho-Oncology, 14,* 875–884. doi:10.1002/pon.947